THRIVING AFTER STROKE

Your Guide to a Fulfilling Life

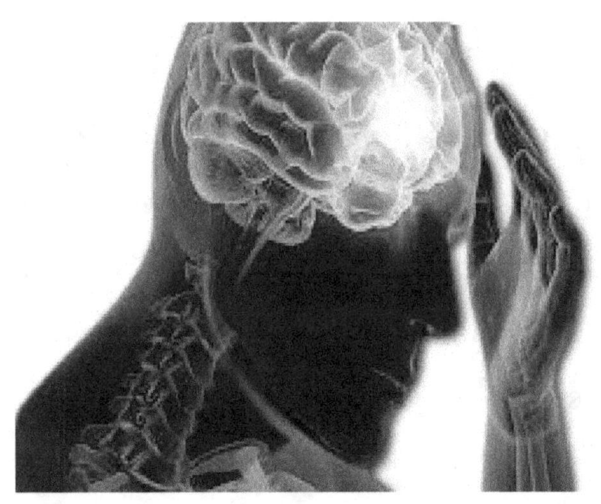

BY: DR. JADEN CLINTON

TABLE OF CONTENT

INTRODUCTION

Visualize waking up one morning to a world turned upside down. That's what experiencing a stroke can feel like. It can leave you speechless, struggling to find the words you once knew so well. It can sap your strength, making a simple walk across the room feel like running a marathon. But here's the incredible truth: a stroke doesn't have to define your life.

Take John, for example. He was a dynamic architect who loved the thrill of scaling buildings as part of his job. When a stroke robbed him of the use of his right arm, it was a crushing blow to his career. Yet, John refused to be sidelined. He taught himself to use design software with his left hand and became a champion for accessibility features. Today, he's not only designing buildings but also making them more inclusive for everyone.

Then there's Sarah, a grandmother whose stroke impaired her speech. She felt frustrated and isolated, almost ready to give up. But Sarah had a secret weapon: her granddaughter, Emily. Together, they embarked on a journey to rediscover communication. Using apps, picture cards, and sheer determination, Sarah rebuilt her voice. Now, she's an iPad whiz, leading online stroke support groups and inspiring others.

John and Sarah are just two of the countless stroke survivors who have defied the odds. This book is your roadmap to join them. It's not about limitations; it's a rallying cry for rebooting your life after a stroke.

Forget about just surviving; it's time to thrive.

We'll inquire into the science behind stroke recovery, but don't worry—this won't be a dry, clinical textbook. We'll break down complex medical jargon into actionable steps you can start taking today. We'll be with you through physical therapy sessions, share laughs as you rediscover forgotten passions, and offer support during the emotional ups and downs.

Most importantly, you won't be alone on this journey. We'll share real-life stories from stroke survivors like John and Sarah, recounting their struggles, victories, and the creative strategies they developed. You'll also hear from medical professionals, therapists, and caregivers, all providing their insights and practical advice.

This book is your guide, your cheerleader, and your toolkit. It's designed to help you reclaim your health, rebuild your independence, and rediscover the fulfilling life that's waiting for you after a stroke. Are you ready to rewrite your story? Let's get started.

CHAPTER ONE

THE STROKE JOURNEY

1.1 WHAT IS A STROKE AND ITS TYPES?

One minute you're making breakfast and planning your day, and the next, everything goes blurry. Your arm feels heavy, your speech slurs, and a strange numbness spreads across your face. It feels like a scene from a bad movie, but this isn't fiction—it's the frightening reality of a stroke.

A stroke occurs when blood flow to part of your brain is interrupted. Just like any other organ, your brain needs a constant supply of oxygen and nutrients, which are delivered through the bloodstream. When this flow is disrupted, brain cells begin to die within minutes. The longer the interruption, the more damage occurs, potentially leading to lasting impairments.

It's a sobering thought, but understanding the different types of strokes is the first step toward regaining control.

Let's explore the two main types: ischemic strokes and hemorrhagic strokes.

The Block Party Gone Wrong: Ischemic Strokes

Imagine your brain as a bustling city, with arteries acting as highways delivering essential supplies. Ischemic strokes occur when a blood clot, like a rogue traffic jam, blocks these highways. This can happen in two primary ways:

Thrombotic stroke: This occurs when a clot forms inside one of the brain's arteries, similar to a slow buildup on a busy road. It's the most common type of ischemic stroke, often caused by conditions like high blood pressure, high cholesterol, and diabetes.

Embolic stroke: Here, a blood clot forms elsewhere in the body, perhaps in the heart, and then travels through the bloodstream until it gets stuck in a narrow brain artery. This is like a piece of debris causing a blockage further down the line.

The Burst Pipe Scenario: Hemorrhagic Strokes

Hemorrhagic strokes are less common but equally dangerous. Instead of a blockage, a weakened blood vessel in the brain ruptures, leading to bleeding in the surrounding tissue. Imagine a burst pipe flooding your apartment—that's the kind of disruption a hemorrhagic stroke causes.

There are two main types of hemorrhagic strokes:

Intracerebral hemorrhage: This is like the main water pipe in your brain bursting, causing widespread damage. It's often linked to uncontrolled high blood pressure or weakened blood vessel walls due to aging or medical conditions.

Subarachnoid hemorrhage: This occurs when a blood vessel on the surface of your brain ruptures, causing bleeding into the space between the brain and the protective membranes that surround it. This type of stroke can cause severe headaches and sometimes seizures.

Recognizing the Signs of a Stroke

Strokes don't come with a warning. They often strike suddenly, leaving you feeling confused and disoriented. However, there are warning signs to watch for. Remember the acronym **FAST**:

- Face: Does one side of your face droop or feel numb?
- Arms: Can you raise both arms equally, or is one arm weak or numb?
- Speech: Is your speech slurred or difficult to understand?
- Time: If you experience any of these symptoms, call emergency services immediately. Time lost is brain lost—the sooner you get medical attention, the better your chances of recovery.

Understanding these signs and acting quickly can make a significant difference. Recognizing a stroke early and getting immediate help is crucial to minimize damage and maximize your chances of recovery.

1.2 Recognizing the Signs and Acting FAST

You never know when life will throw you a curveball. One moment you're laughing with a friend, and the next, something feels off. Maybe your arm feels heavy, your speech slurs, or the world seems tilted. It feels like a scene from a movie, but this is real—this could be a stroke.

The good news? Strokes often give us warning signs, precious moments to act before the damage becomes severe. But the window of opportunity is narrow. That's where the acronym FAST comes in—a lifesaving tool that can make all the difference in your recovery journey.

Face: The Drop of Disruption

Imagine trying to smile, but only one side of your face moves. This is a classic sign of a stroke—facial drooping or numbness. A stroke can disrupt the nerve signals controlling your facial muscles. Look in the mirror: can you raise both eyebrows equally? Does one side of your mouth droop when you try to smile? Ask a friend or family member to observe you—sometimes, we might not notice these subtle changes ourselves.

Arms: Weakness Takes the Lead

Imagine reaching for a cup of coffee, but one arm feels heavy or numb. This is another red flag for a stroke. A stroke can weaken the muscles on one side of your body, making it difficult to raise both arms with equal strength. Here's a simple test: with your eyes closed, try raising both arms straight out in front of you. Does one arm drift downward? This could be a sign of weakness and requires immediate medical attention.

Speech: The Lost Words

Imagine struggling to form words, your speech slurred or garbled. This can happen because a stroke can affect the areas of the brain responsible for language production and comprehension. Does your speech sound strange to you or others? Are you having trouble finding the right words or forming complete sentences? Don't hesitate to seek help if you experience any sudden changes in your speech patterns.

Time: Don't Wait, Act Now!

This is perhaps the most crucial aspect of FAST. Time lost is brain lost. Every minute a stroke goes untreated, millions of brain cells die. Don't wait for symptoms to disappear or convince yourself it's "just a headache." If you suspect a stroke in yourself or someone around you, call emergency services immediately. Even if the symptoms seem mild or come and go, err on the side of caution.

Beyond FAST: Additional Warning Signs

While FAST covers the most common symptoms, strokes can manifest in different ways. Here are some additional signs to be aware of:

Sudden severe headache: A sudden, excruciating headache can be a sign of a hemorrhagic stroke caused by bleeding in the brain.

Vision problems: Sudden blurred or double vision, or even complete vision loss in one eye, can be a stroke symptom.

Dizziness, loss of balance, or coordination problems: Feeling unsteady, lightheaded, or having difficulty walking or maintaining balance could indicate a stroke.

The Importance of Acting FAST: A Story of Survival

Envisage Barbara, a vibrant grandmother enjoying a walk with her grandchildren. Suddenly, she feels a strange numbness in her right arm. Dismissing it as a muscle cramp, she continues walking. But then her speech becomes slurred, and she struggles to form words. Panicked, her grandchildren recognize the signs and immediately call emergency services.

Thanks to their quick action and Barbara's knowledge of FAST, she received medical attention within the crucial timeframe. After undergoing treatment, Barbara made a remarkable recovery, regaining most of her motor skills and speech abilities. Her story is a testament to the power of recognizing stroke symptoms and acting FAST.

1.3 The Immediate Aftermath: Treatment and Hospitalization

The world feels upside down. You've just had a stroke, and the initial shock and fear are overwhelming. But amid the confusion, there's a flicker of hope—you've received medical attention, and your recovery journey has begun. Now, you're facing a new challenge: navigating the hospital environment and the whirlwind of tests and treatments.

This chapter will be your guide, helping you through the immediate aftermath of a stroke. We'll cover what to expect during hospitalization, the various treatment options available, and how to be an active participant in your recovery.

The Emergency Room Frenzy: Initial Assessment and Stabilization

Picture yourself arriving at the emergency room, the atmosphere buzzing with activity. Doctors and nurses will work quickly to assess your condition, which may involve several tests, including:

- Blood tests: To check blood sugar levels, clotting factors, and signs of infection.

- Brain imaging: CT scans or MRIs to determine the location and type of stroke.

- Electrocardiogram (ECG): To check your heart rhythm and identify potential sources of blood clots.

The primary goal in the emergency room is to stabilize your condition and minimize brain damage. Depending on the type of stroke, treatment options might include:

Thrombolytic therapy (clot-busting drugs): Administered intravenously within a critical timeframe (usually 3-4.5 hours) to dissolve blood clots and restore blood flow to the brain.

Endovascular thrombectomy: A minimally invasive procedure where a catheter is inserted into an artery to remove the clot directly.

Blood pressure control: Medications to lower high blood pressure, which can further damage brain tissue.

Surgery: In some cases, surgery may be necessary to remove a large blood clot or repair a bleeding blood vessel.

Finding Your Footing: Life in the Hospital

After initial stabilization, you'll likely be admitted to a specialized stroke unit for further observation and treatment. This unit is staffed by medical professionals with expertise in stroke care, providing a comprehensive approach to your recovery. Here's what you can expect:

Monitoring vital signs: Your blood pressure, heart rate, and oxygen levels will be closely monitored.

Medication management: You'll continue receiving medications to control blood pressure, cholesterol, and prevent future blood clots.

Physical and occupational therapy: Therapists will help you regain mobility, improve coordination, and relearn daily skills like eating, dressing, and bathing.

Speech and language therapy: If your stroke affected your speech or communication abilities, therapists will help you develop strategies to regain your voice and improve communication skills.

Becoming an Active Participant in Your Recovery

Remember, you're not just a patient; you're an active participant in your recovery journey. Here's how you can take charge:

Ask questions: Don't hesitate to ask your doctors and nurses about your diagnosis, treatment plan, and potential risks and benefits.

Be an advocate for yourself: Clearly communicate your needs and concerns to your healthcare team.

Start small, celebrate big: Celebrate small improvements in mobility, speech, or coordination.

Focus on a positive mindset: Recovery takes time and effort. Maintaining a positive outlook can strengthen your resilience and improve long-term outcomes.

While the hospital environment might seem daunting, remember, it's a safe haven where you can focus on healing. The dedicated medical team is there to guide you every step of the way.

Beyond the Hospital Walls: Preparing for Discharge

As you near discharge, the hospital staff will work with you to develop a comprehensive discharge plan. This plan might include:

Rehabilitation options: Continuing outpatient rehabilitation therapy to further improve your functional skills.

Medications: Prescriptions to manage your health conditions and prevent future strokes.

Home modifications: Recommendations to modify your home environment to ensure safety and accessibility.

Support groups: Connecting with other stroke survivors for emotional support and encouragement on your recovery journey.

The road to recovery from a stroke is unique for everyone. While the initial phase in the hospital sets the stage for healing, it's just the beginning. In the following chapters, we'll delve deeper into the journey of regaining your strength and independence, exploring physical therapy techniques, managing cognitive challenges, and adopting a healthy lifestyle for long-term well-being.

CHAPTER TWO

THE IMPACT OF STROKE

2.1 PHYSICAL CHANGES AND POTENTIAL CHALLENGES

Imagine waking up in a hospital bed, everything looking slightly off-kilter. Your arm feels heavy, your speech is slurred, and lifting a glass of water seems like a herculean task. These are the harsh realities of the physical changes following a stroke. While the initial shock might leave you feeling discouraged, remember this: your body has an incredible capacity for healing. This chapter will guide you through the potential physical changes you might encounter after a stroke and equip you with strategies to rebuild your strength and reclaim your independence.

The Stroke's Impact: A Mosaic of Challenges

Strokes affect different parts of the brain, and the physical consequences can vary greatly from person to person.

Here's a breakdown of some common challenges you might face:

Weakness or Paralysis: This is one of the most frequent consequences of a stroke. Depending on the affected area of the brain, you might experience weakness or complete paralysis on one side of your body, making activities like walking, dressing, and self-care difficult. This is often referred to as hemiparesis (weakness) or hemiplegia (paralysis).

Spasticity and Stiffness: Muscles on the affected side of your body might become stiff and tight, making movement painful and limiting your range of motion.

Loss of Coordination and Balance: A stroke can affect your coordination and balance, increasing your risk of falls. Simple tasks like reaching for an object or walking on uneven surfaces might become challenging.

Sensory Changes: You might experience numbness, tingling, or burning sensations on the affected side of your body, making activities like walking or dressing uncomfortable and disorienting.

Fatigue: Recovering from a stroke takes a lot of energy. You might experience fatigue and exhaustion, making it difficult to participate in rehabilitation activities for extended periods.

These physical changes can be incredibly frustrating and significantly impact your daily life. But remember, this isn't the end of the story.

The Power of Rehabilitation: Your Path to Recovery

Physical and occupational therapy will be your guiding light on the road to recovery. Therapists will work with you to design a personalized rehabilitation program that addresses your specific needs and goals. Here's what you can expect:

Strengthening Exercises: These exercises aim to improve muscle strength and coordination on the affected side of your body. They might involve using weights, resistance bands, or your own body weight.

Range of Motion Exercises: These exercises help loosen tight muscles and improve your flexibility, making daily activities more manageable.

Balance and Gait Training: Therapists will work with you to improve your balance and coordination, reducing your risk of falls. This might involve using specialized equipment or practicing walking on different surfaces.

Activities of Daily Living (ADL) Training: Therapists will help you relearn essential skills like dressing, bathing, and toileting, promoting your independence in daily life.

Assistive Devices: Depending on your needs, therapists might recommend assistive devices like canes, walkers, or grab bars to help you move around safely and independently.

Beyond Therapy: Strategies for Everyday Life

Rehabilitation is just one piece of the puzzle. Here are some additional tips to help you manage physical changes after a stroke and promote your recovery:

Pacing Yourself: Don't try to do too much too soon. Listen to your body and take breaks when you get tired.

Staying Active: Incorporate light physical activity into your daily routine, even if it's just a short walk around your house. Regular exercise can improve your strength, stamina, and overall well-being.

Maintaining Good Posture: Proper posture can help prevent pain and muscle stiffness. Therapists can teach you specific techniques to maintain good posture while sitting, standing, and walking.

Healthy Eating: A balanced diet rich in fruits, vegetables, and whole grains provides your body with the nutrients needed for healing and recovery.

Staying Hydrated: Drinking plenty of water helps your body function optimally and can help prevent fatigue.

The Road Ahead: Embracing Patience and Perseverance

Recovery from a stroke is a marathon, not a sprint. There will be setbacks and days when progress seems slow. But with patience, perseverance, and a dedicated team by your side, you can rebuild your strength, regain your independence, and live a fulfilling life after a stroke.

2.2 Emotional and Mental Health After Stroke

Picture the emotional turmoil you might experience after a stroke. One minute you're brimming with confidence, the next, you're frustrated because buttoning your shirt feels impossible. It's a rollercoaster of emotions – anger, sadness, fear, and a sense of isolation. These are all valid responses to the dramatic changes brought on by a stroke. But here's the good news: you're not alone in this emotional journey, and there are strategies to help you navigate the highs and lows.

The Emotional Landscape After Stroke

A stroke doesn't just affect the physical body; it can significantly impact your emotional and mental well-being. Here are some common emotional challenges you might encounter:

Depression: The sudden loss of independence and the challenges of recovery can trigger feelings of sadness, hopelessness, and worthlessness.

Anxiety: The fear of another stroke, uncertainty about the future, and frustration over limitations can lead to anxiety and panic attacks.

Anger and Frustration: The inability to do things you once took for granted can be incredibly frustrating, leading to outbursts of anger or irritability.

Grief and Loss: You might grieve the loss of your previous abilities, your sense of self, or the life you envisioned before the stroke.

Social Isolation: Emotional challenges can lead to social withdrawal, resulting in feelings of isolation and loneliness.

The Fog of Change: Addressing Cognitive Challenges

Beyond emotions, a stroke can also affect your cognitive abilities. Here are some potential challenges you might face:

Memory Problems: Difficulty remembering recent events, forgetting names or faces, or struggling to learn new information.

Concentration Difficulties: Trouble focusing on tasks, getting easily distracted, or difficulty completing multi-step activities.

Problem-Solving Challenges: Difficulty making decisions, planning activities, or following complex instructions.

Communication Problems: Difficulty finding the right words, slurred speech, or difficulty understanding what others are saying.

These cognitive changes can be incredibly frustrating, making it difficult to return to work or engage in activities you once enjoyed. But there are ways to manage them.

Finding Your Compass: Strategies for Emotional and Mental Well-being

Navigating the emotional and mental challenges after a stroke requires a multi-pronged approach. Here are some strategies to help you cope:

Acknowledge Your Emotions: Don't bottle up your feelings. Talk to a therapist, counselor, or support group about what you're experiencing. It's okay to feel sad, frustrated, or angry.

Join a Support Group: Connecting with other stroke survivors can provide invaluable emotional support and a sense of community. Knowing you're not alone can make a big difference.

Practice Relaxation Techniques: Techniques like deep breathing, meditation, and mindfulness can help manage stress and anxiety.

Seek Professional Help: If you're struggling to cope emotionally, don't hesitate to seek professional help from a therapist or counselor. They can equip you with strategies for managing depression, anxiety, and other challenges.

Cognitive Rehabilitation: Therapists can help you develop strategies to improve your memory, concentration, and problem-solving skills.

Taking Care of Yourself: Prioritizing Mental Well-being

Just like your physical health, your mental health needs attention too. Here are some self-care tips to promote your overall well-being:

Get Enough Sleep: Adequate sleep allows your brain to rest and recover, which can improve your mood and cognitive function.

Eat a Healthy Diet: A balanced diet rich in fruits, vegetables, and whole grains provides your brain with the nutrients it needs to function optimally.

Stay Active: Regular exercise releases endorphins, natural mood boosters that can combat depression and anxiety.

Engage in Activities You Enjoy: Don't give up on things you love to do. Find ways to adapt them to your new abilities or explore new activities that bring you joy.

The Road to Acceptance and Renewal

Coming to terms with the emotional and mental changes after a stroke takes time. There will be good days and bad days. But remember, acceptance is not giving up; it's about acknowledging your challenges and finding ways to move forward. With dedication, self-care, and the support of your healthcare team and loved ones, you can navigate the emotional rollercoaster and reclaim your mental well-being.

2.3 Addressing Communication Difficulties

Imagine reaching for the phone to call a friend, only to find your words tangled in your mind. Frustration builds as you struggle to form a sentence, and the simplest conversation feels like climbing a mountain. Communication difficulties are a common consequence of stroke, robbing you of the ability to express yourself clearly and connect with others. But here's the inspiring truth: with the right strategies and a little perseverance, you can regain your voice and rebuild your communication skills.

The Spectrum of Communication Challenges

Strokes can affect different areas of the brain responsible for communication, leading to various challenges. Here's a breakdown of some common difficulties you might encounter:

Aphasia: This is perhaps the most well-known communication difficulty after a stroke. It can manifest in different ways, including:

Expressive aphasia: Difficulty finding the right words to express yourself, leading to frustration and a feeling of being trapped in your own mind.

Receptive aphasia: Difficulty understanding what others are saying, making conversations confusing and disorienting.

Anomic aphasia: Difficulty remembering names of objects or people, making communication frustrating for both you and the listener.

Dysarthria: This affects the muscles involved in speech production, making it difficult to speak clearly or control the volume and pace of your speech. Words might come out slurred, mumbled, or strained.

Apraxia of speech: Difficulty coordinating the movements of your lips, tongue, and vocal cords to form sounds and words. This can lead to speech that is hesitant, slow, and effortful.

Finding Your Voice Again: Speech and Language Therapy

Speech and language therapy will be your guiding light on the path to regaining your communication skills. Therapists will work with you to assess your specific challenges and develop a personalized therapy plan. Here's what you can expect:

Speech exercises: Therapists will guide you through exercises to strengthen the muscles involved in speech production, improving your articulation and clarity.

Language stimulation activities: These activities aim to improve your vocabulary, comprehension skills, and ability to find the right words.

Communication strategies: Therapists will teach you techniques to compensate for your communication difficulties. This might involve using gestures, pictures, or communication apps to supplement your spoken words.

Alternative and Augmentative Communication (AAC) devices: Depending on your needs, therapists might introduce you to AAC devices like voice synthesizers or picture boards to help you express yourself effectively.

Beyond Therapy: Strategies for Everyday Communication

Speech therapy equips you with tools, but you'll also need practical strategies for everyday communication. Here are some tips to help you navigate conversations:

Be patient: Communication takes time and effort after a stroke. Don't get discouraged if progress feels slow.

Speak slowly and clearly: This can help the listener understand your words better.

Use short sentences and simple language: This can make conversations less overwhelming.

- Don't be afraid to ask for clarification: If you don't understand something, politely ask the person to rephrase it.

- Use gestures and facial expressions: This can add context and meaning to your words.

- Practice, practice, practice: The more you communicate, the stronger your skills will become.

The Power of Patience and Support

Communication difficulties can be incredibly frustrating, but remember, you're not alone in this journey. Here are some additional tips to navigate this challenge:

Involve your family and friends: Educate your loved ones about your communication difficulties and enlist their support. They can be patient listeners and help you find alternative ways to express yourself.

Join a support group: Connecting with other stroke survivors who have communication challenges can provide valuable emotional support and a sense of community.

Celebrate small victories: Don't wait for grand achievements. Celebrate every small improvement in your communication skills, no matter how big or small.

Technology to the Rescue: Tools and Apps for Communication

Technology offers a helping hand in overcoming communication challenges. Here are some tools and apps to explore:

Speech recognition software: These programs can transcribe your spoken words into text, allowing you to communicate via email or messaging apps.

Text-to-speech software: These programs can convert written text into spoken words, allowing you to "speak" through a synthesized voice.

Augmentative and Alternative Communication (AAC) apps: These apps provide a variety of tools and symbols to help you communicate your needs and wants, even if you have difficulty speaking.

The Road to Connection: Finding Your Voice Again

Regaining your communication skills after a stroke takes time, dedication, and a supportive network. But with the right strategies, technology, and perseverance, you can find your voice again and rebuild your ability to connect with others. Remember, every small step forward is a victory worth celebrating.

CHAPTER THREE

BUILDING YOUR CARE TEAM

3.1 PARTNERING WITH DOCTORS AND SPECIALISTS

After a stroke, the hospital can feel like a whirlwind of activity – tests, scans, medications, and a constant stream of medical professionals. It can be overwhelming, but remember, this team is on your side. Doctors, nurses, therapists, and specialists all play a crucial role in your recovery journey. Here, we'll delve into the importance of building a strong partnership with your healthcare team and maximizing the benefits of each specialist's expertise.

Your Stroke Care Team: A harmony of Expertise

Think of your stroke care team as an orchestra, with each member playing a vital role in the symphony of your recovery. Here are some key players you might encounter:

Neurologist: Specializes in the nervous system, including the brain. They diagnose the type of stroke you've had, determine the cause, and develop a long-term treatment plan to prevent future strokes.

Physiatrist: A rehabilitation specialist who works alongside physical and occupational therapists to create a personalized therapy program that helps you regain lost mobility and independence.

Physical Therapist: Focuses on improving your muscle strength, coordination, and balance, allowing you to perform daily activities like walking, dressing, and bathing.

Occupational Therapist: Helps you relearn essential skills for daily living, such as managing your home environment, preparing meals, or returning to work.

Speech-Language Pathologist: If you have communication difficulties like aphasia or dysarthria, this therapist will work with you to improve your speech, language skills, and swallowing abilities.

Cardiologist: Manages your heart health if your stroke is linked to heart problems like arrhythmia or high blood pressure, reducing the risk of future strokes.

Social Worker: Provides resources and support to help you navigate the emotional and social challenges of recovery. They can also connect you with support groups and community services.

Building a Strong Partnership: Communication is Key

Having a strong, collaborative relationship with your healthcare team is essential for a successful recovery. Here's how to ensure effective communication:

Ask questions: Don't hesitate to ask about your diagnosis, treatment plan, potential side effects, and long-term outlook. Knowledge empowers you to be an active participant in your recovery.

Express your concerns: If you have any worries about your medications, therapy sessions, or overall health, voice them clearly to your doctor.

Bring a notebook to appointments: Take notes during appointments to record important information, medications, and follow-up instructions.

Advocate for yourself: Be your own health advocate. Don't be afraid to ask for clarification or seek a second opinion if you feel something isn't right.

Maintain open communication: Share any changes in your health, medication schedules, or emotional well-being with your doctors.

Maximizing Each Specialist's Expertise: Getting the Most Out of Your Appointments

To get the most out of your appointments with different specialists, here are some tips:

Come prepared: Write down any questions you have beforehand to ensure you cover all your concerns during the limited appointment time.

Gather relevant information: Bring a list of medications you're currently taking, any recent medical reports or test results, and information about any past medical conditions.

Be specific about your challenges: When working with therapists, be specific about the difficulties you're facing in daily activities. This helps them tailor their therapy program to your needs.

Actively participate in discussions: Don't be a passive listener. Share your experiences, goals, and challenges openly with your healthcare team.

The Power of Collaboration: Working Together for Optimal Results

Building a strong partnership with your doctors and specialists is a two-way street. When you actively participate in your care, communicate openly, and leverage the expertise of each team member, the results can be truly transformative. This collaborative approach allows your healthcare team to:

Develop a comprehensive treatment plan: By considering the input from various specialists, your doctors can create a holistic plan that addresses all aspects of your recovery, from physical rehabilitation to emotional well-being.

Monitor your progress effectively: Regular check-ins with each specialist allow them to track your progress, identify any potential complications, and adjust your treatment plan as needed.

Provide ongoing support: Your healthcare team is there for you in the long run. They can offer guidance and support as you transition back to work, manage your health at home, and prevent future strokes.

Beyond the Doctor's Office: Building a Support Network

Your healthcare team is a crucial component of your recovery, but they're not the only ones on your side. Building a strong support network of family, friends, and fellow stroke survivors can make a world of difference in your emotional well-being and overall success on your recovery journey. Here's how to expand your support circle:

Involve your family and friends: Educate your loved ones about stroke and its effects. Explain your limitations, be open about your challenges, and enlist their support in daily activities.

Seek out a support group: Connecting with other stroke survivors can be incredibly empowering. Sharing experiences, learning from each other's triumphs and struggles, and gaining emotional support can significantly boost your morale.

Consider online communities: Online forums and social media groups specifically for stroke survivors can be a source of information, encouragement, and connection with others who understand your journey.

The Role of Family and Friends: A Circle of Strength

Your family and friends are your first line of support. Here's how to strengthen this bond:

Be open and honest: Communicate your needs and limitations clearly. This allows them to offer support in ways that are truly helpful.

Delegate tasks: Don't be afraid to ask for help with errands, chores, or transportation. Sharing responsibilities reduces your burden and allows your loved ones to feel involved.

Maintain open communication: Talk about your feelings, frustrations, and anxieties. Supportive friends and family can be a source of comfort and understanding.

Finding Your Tribe: The Power of Support Groups

Support groups offer a unique kind of camaraderie. Here's how to find and benefit from them:

Ask your doctor or therapist: They might be aware of stroke support groups in your area.

Search online resources: Many stroke organizations maintain online databases of support groups across the country.

Consider online groups: If in-person meetings are difficult, online support groups can be a valuable alternative.

Be open to sharing: Don't be afraid to share your experiences and challenges. Your story might resonate with others and offer them comfort and support.

The Road to Resilience: Building a Life After Stroke

Recovery from a stroke is a marathon, not a sprint. There will be setbacks and days when progress feels slow. But with a strong healthcare team by your side, a supportive network of loved ones, and a never-give-up attitude, you can rebuild your life after a stroke. The next chapter will delve into the importance of a healthy lifestyle in preventing future strokes and promoting long-term well-being. We'll explore strategies for managing risk factors, adopting a healthy diet, and incorporating regular exercise into your routine. Remember, you're not just healing from a stroke; you're building the foundation for a healthier, happier you.

3.2 The Role of Therapists and Rehabilitation

In the aftermath of a stroke, regaining your lost abilities can seem overwhelming. But there is hope. Rehabilitation, guided by a dedicated team of therapists, will be your compass on the road to recovery. These skilled professionals will help you rebuild your strength, improve your mobility, and rediscover your independence. Let's explore the different types of therapists you might encounter and the crucial role they play in your recovery journey.

The Rehabilitation Team: Your Allies in Healing

Rehabilitation is a collaborative effort. Here are some key therapists you'll likely work with:

Physical Therapist: Focuses on improving your physical abilities. They design exercises to strengthen muscles, enhance coordination, and improve balance. Their goal is to help you regain mobility and control over your body, enabling you to perform daily activities like walking, dressing, and bathing.

Occupational Therapist: Helps you relearn essential skills for daily living. They assess your home environment and recommend modifications for safety and independence. They also help you practice tasks like cooking, managing finances, or returning to work.

Speech-Language Pathologist: If you have communication difficulties like aphasia or dysarthria, this therapist will work with you to improve your speech, language skills, and swallowing abilities. They develop strategies to help you express yourself effectively and navigate communication challenges.

Cognitive Rehabilitation Therapist: Focuses on improving cognitive skills affected by the stroke, such as memory, attention, and problem-solving. They develop exercises and strategies to enhance these abilities and help you compensate for any cognitive challenges.

A Tailored Approach: Building Your Rehabilitation Program

There's no one-size-fits-all approach to rehabilitation. Your therapist will conduct a comprehensive assessment to understand your specific needs and goals. Based on this assessment, they will create a personalized rehabilitation program that addresses your unique challenges. This program might include:

Physical Exercises: Designed to improve muscle strength, coordination, and balance. These might involve weights, resistance bands, or bodyweight exercises, with increasing intensity as you progress.

Balance and Gait Training: Therapists will work with you to improve balance and coordination, reducing your risk of falls. This might involve practicing walking on different surfaces or using specialized equipment.

Activities of Daily Living (ADL) Training: Therapists will help you relearn essential skills for daily living, such as dressing, bathing, and toileting. They can recommend assistive devices like canes, walkers, or grab bars to promote your independence.

Communication Therapy: For those with communication difficulties, therapists work to improve speech clarity, vocabulary, and comprehension. They might also teach alternative communication methods like picture boards or communication apps.

Cognitive Retraining Exercises: These exercises aim to improve cognitive skills like memory, attention, and problem-solving, using tools such as memory games, puzzles, or computer-based programs.

Beyond Exercises: The Importance of Therapy Sessions

While exercises are crucial, rehabilitation is more than just physical training. Therapy sessions also provide a safe space to:

Express Concerns and Frustrations: Therapists can be a listening ear and offer emotional support as you navigate the challenges of recovery.

Learn Coping Strategies: Therapists can teach strategies for managing pain, fatigue, and emotional challenges that might accompany stroke.

Set Realistic Goals: Working with your therapist, you can set achievable goals for your recovery, keeping you motivated and on track.

Celebrate Achievements: Rehabilitation is a journey of small victories. Therapists will celebrate your progress, no matter how big or small, fostering a sense of accomplishment and boosting your morale.

Building a Strong Therapist-Patient Relationship

A strong relationship with your therapist is essential for a successful recovery. Here's how to nurture this connection:

Be Open and Honest: Communicate openly about your limitations, goals, and any challenges you're facing.

Ask Questions: Don't hesitate to ask questions about your exercises, treatment plan, or any concerns you might have.

Be an Active Participant: Actively participate in your therapy sessions and complete your exercises diligently at home.

Provide Feedback: Let your therapist know if you're struggling with certain exercises or if the program needs adjustments.

The Road to Independence: Partnering for Long-Term Success

Rehabilitation doesn't end when you leave the therapy clinic. Therapists will equip you with the tools and strategies to continue your recovery journey at home. They can also connect you with resources and support groups to ensure long-term success.

With the support of your rehabilitation team and a strong commitment to your recovery, you can overcome the challenges posed by a stroke and build a healthier, more independent life.

3.3 Building a Support System: Family, Friends, and Caregivers

The road to recovery after a stroke is rarely traveled alone. While medical professionals play a crucial role in your rehabilitation, having a strong support system of family, friends, and caregivers is equally important for your emotional well-being and long-term success. This network provides encouragement, practical assistance, and a sense of belonging as you navigate the challenges and triumphs of your recovery.

The Pillars of Support: Family and Friends

Your family and friends are often the first to step in after a stroke. Here's how to make the most of their love and support:

Open Communication: Be honest with your loved ones about the physical and emotional challenges you're facing. Explain your limitations and clearly communicate your needs.

Educate Your Circle: Help your family and friends understand stroke, its effects, and your recovery process.

This knowledge enables them to support you in meaningful ways.

Delegate Tasks: Don't hesitate to ask for help with errands, chores, or transportation. Sharing responsibilities reduces your burden and lets your loved ones feel involved.

Maintain Open Communication: Share your feelings, frustrations, and anxieties. Supportive friends and family can provide comfort, understanding, and a listening ear.

Celebrate Milestones: Celebrate your victories, no matter how big or small, with your loved ones. Their encouragement will boost your morale and keep you motivated.

Finding the Right Caregiver: When Additional Support is Needed

Sometimes, you might need extra support beyond what family and friends can provide. Here's how to find the right caregiver:

Assess Your Needs: Identify the areas where you need the most help, such as daily living activities, medication management, or transportation.

Consider Different Options: Explore various caregiver options, such as professional home care agencies, private caregivers, or family members who can take on a more active caregiving role.

Interview Potential Caregivers: When interviewing potential caregivers, assess their experience, qualifications, and personality. Choose someone you feel comfortable with and who understands your specific needs.

Communicate Clearly: Clearly outline your expectations and needs to your caregiver. This ensures they can provide the best possible support.

Maintain Open Communication: Keep an open line of communication with your caregiver. Discuss any concerns or challenges and work together to create a supportive care plan.

Beyond Practical Help: The Emotional Support System

Your support system extends beyond practical help to provide crucial emotional support:

A Listening Ear: Having someone to listen without judgment can be invaluable.

A Source of Encouragement: Supportive friends and family can be your biggest cheerleaders, motivating you during tough times and celebrating your successes.

A Sense of Belonging: Feeling connected to loved ones can combat the isolation and loneliness that sometimes accompany stroke recovery.

A Partner in Advocacy: Family and friends can help you navigate medical appointments, insurance issues, and access necessary resources.

Building a Strong Support Network: Tips for Success

Here are some tips for building an effective support network:

Be Patient: Building a strong support system takes time. Be patient with yourself and your loved ones as you adjust to the new normal.

Set Boundaries: It's okay to set boundaries. Communicate your needs clearly and respectfully.

Express Gratitude: Don't forget to express appreciation for the love and support you receive from your family, friends, and caregivers.

The Ripple Effect of Support: A Network of Strength

A strong support system isn't just about receiving help; it's also about giving back. As you progress in your recovery, consider offering support to others facing similar challenges. Sharing your experiences and offering encouragement can create a ripple effect of strength within your community.

CHAPTER FOUR

RESTORING MOBILITY

4.1 PHYSICAL THERAPY: EXERCISES FOR REGAINING MUSCLE CONTROL

After a stroke, getting back control over your muscles is a big step towards recovery. Physical therapy is key here, and your therapist will tailor exercises just for you, focusing on your needs and limitations. Let's take a look at some common exercises used in physical therapy to boost muscle strength, coordination, and balance post-stroke.

Important Reminder: Before diving into any new exercise routine, always check in with your doctor or physical therapist. They'll make sure the exercises are safe and suitable for you.

Strengthening Exercises for Major Muscle Groups

Let's break down some exercises that target major muscle groups and can be adjusted based on your abilities:

Upper Body Strength:

1. Arm Raises: Sit or stand tall, holding weights or water bottles. Lift your arms out to the sides until they're parallel to the floor, then lower them slowly. Repeat 10-12 times.

2. Bicep Curls: With weights in hand, bend your elbows, bringing the weights towards your shoulders. Repeat 10-12 times.

3. Triceps Extensions: Hold weights overhead, then bend your elbows, lowering the weights behind your head. Straighten your elbows to lift them back up. Repeat 10-12 times.

Lower Body Strength:

1. Squats: Stand with feet shoulder-width apart, lower yourself as if sitting in a chair, then stand back up. Repeat 10-12 times.

2. Leg Extensions: Sit and extend one leg straight out with a resistance band around your ankle. Repeat 10-12 times for each leg.

3. Calf Raises: Stand and rise onto your toes, then slowly lower your heels back down. Repeat 10-12 times.

Coordination Exercises for Movement Control

Good coordination is key for daily tasks. Try these exercises to enhance your movement control:

1. Heel-to-Toe Walking: Walk heel-to-toe in a straight line, focusing on balance.

2. Reaching Exercises: Stand with feet shoulder-width apart, reach forward to touch the floor while keeping your back straight. Repeat with each arm.

3. Ball Transfers: Sit with two objects on a table, transfer them between hands. Focus on controlled movements.

Balance Exercises to Find Your Footing

Maintaining balance helps prevent falls. Here are exercises to improve your balance:

1. Single Leg Stance: Stand with support, lift one leg off the ground, hold, then switch legs. Progress to standing without support.

2. Walking on Different Surfaces: Practice walking on grass, carpet, or uneven ground to challenge your balance.

Tips for Making Therapy Work for You

Maximize the benefits of your therapy sessions with these tips:

1. Active Participation: Get involved, ask questions, and communicate your needs and concerns.

2. Practice at Home: Reinforce what you learn in therapy by practicing at home regularly.

3. Set Realistic Goals: Work with your therapist to set achievable goals and celebrate milestones along the way.

Adapting Exercises for Home Practice

You can adapt many therapy exercises for home practice using everyday items:

1. Ankle weights: Use soup cans filled with beans for homemade weights.

2. Resistance bands: Mimic therapy bands with elastic bands of varying resistance.

3. Therapy balls: Use a small yoga ball for balance or core exercises.

4. Soup cans: Substitute dumbbells with soup cans for arm exercises.

Enlisting Support from Loved Ones

Involve your family and friends in your therapy journey:

1. Ask for Help: Don't hesitate to ask for assistance or encouragement during home practice.

2. Educate Your Support System: Briefly explain your exercises so they can offer better support.

3. Celebrate Together: Share your progress and victories with loved ones to stay motivated.

Remember, regaining muscle control after a stroke is a journey. Be patient, celebrate small wins, and trust your therapist's guidance. The next chapter will explore the importance of a healthy diet in stroke recovery, focusing on creating a heart-healthy, stroke-preventive diet plan.

4.2 Adapting Your Home for Safe Movement

Reclaiming your home after a stroke can feel like maneuvering an obstacle course, but fret not! With a few adjustments, you can turn your living space into a haven that promotes your recovery and independence. Let's dive into some practical strategies for adapting your home to ensure safe movement and reduce the risk of falls.

Putting Safety First: A Holistic Approach

After a stroke, safety at home is paramount. Here are some areas to focus on:

Fall Prevention: Falls are a major concern post-stroke. We'll look at how to minimize fall risks.

Enhanced Accessibility: Easy access to all parts of your home boosts independence and mobility.

Assistive Devices: Tools like grab bars and walkers can greatly improve safety and comfort.

Ample Lighting: Good lighting is essential for spotting hazards and moving around safely.

PREVENTING FALLS: SECURING YOUR SPACE

Avoiding falls is crucial. Here's how to make your home fall-proof:

Declutter: Keep walkways and floors clear to prevent tripping hazards.

Rug Security: Secure loose rugs with tape or remove them from high-traffic areas.

Bathroom Safety: Install grab bars and consider a bath seat for added stability.

Brighten Up: Ensure your home is well-lit, especially in hallways and bathrooms.

Smooth Surfaces: Repair any uneven floors or steps that could cause trips.

Enhancing Accessibility: Navigating Your Home with Ease

MAKE YOUR HOME EASIER TO NAVIGATE WITH THESE TIPS:

Wider Doorways: Consider widening doorways for wheelchair or walker access.

Accessible Storage: Rearrange cabinets to keep frequently used items within reach.

Lever Handles: Replace doorknobs with lever handles for easier use.

Raised Furniture: Raise chair heights for easier sitting and standing.

Kitchen Tweaks: Lower countertops and add pull-out drawers for easier access.

ASSISTED LIVING: TOOLS FOR MOBILITY

Assistive devices can be game-changers:

Grab Bars: Install them in key areas like bathrooms and stairways for added support.

Walkers or Canes: Use these aids for stability while walking.

Shower Seats: A stable seat in the shower makes bathing safer.

Raised Toilet Seat: Makes sitting and standing easier.

Reacher's: Handy for grabbing objects without bending or straining.

Shedding Light on Safety: Illuminating Your Space

Good lighting is your ally against falls:

- Layered Lighting: Mix overhead and task lighting for a well-lit home.
- Nightlights: Add dimmable nightlights for nighttime safety.
- Contrast Lighting: Opt for high-contrast lighting in critical areas like stairs.
- Adjustable Brightness: Choose fixtures with adjustable brightness to suit your needs.

Creating a safe home is a group effort:

Brainstorm Together: Discuss modifications with family and friends for valuable input.

Delegate Tasks: Get help from capable loved ones, especially for hands-on tasks.

Professional Advice: Consult an occupational therapist for tailored recommendations.

Financial Support: Explore assistance programs to help with modification costs.

Embracing Safety and Independence

Making your home safer post-stroke is a journey, not a sprint. Start with the essentials and adapt as needed. A safe, accessible environment empowers you to live life with confidence and independence. In the next chapter, we'll explore the vital role of a healthy diet in stroke recovery.

4.3 Assistive Devices: Canes, Walkers, and Beyond

Recovering mobility after a stroke is pivotal for your journey back to wellness. Assistive devices can be your trusty companions, offering support, stability, and confidence as you navigate your surroundings. Let's explore some common devices post-stroke, along with tips on selecting the right one for you and using it safely.

Understanding Your Needs: Where to Begin

Your unique needs shape the choice of your device. Consider factors like:

Stroke Severity: The extent of your stroke affects your mobility and support requirements.

Balance and Coordination: If these are challenges, you might need a device offering more stability.

Strength and Endurance: Your physical capabilities determine the type of device suitable for you.

Daily Activities: Think about which tasks, like walking or bathing, you need assistance with.

The Big Three: Canes, Walkers, and Wheelchairs

These are staples in post-stroke mobility aids:

Canes: Provide single-point support, ideal for mild balance issues. Types include standard, offset, and tripod.

Walkers: Offer more support, suited for those needing assistance with balance and walking. Types range from standard to rolling.

Wheelchairs: Essential for those unable to walk independently. Manual, electric, and specialized options are available.

Choosing the Right Device: Getting it Right

Proper fitting is key for comfort and safety:

Consult a therapist: Let your therapist recommend the best device for your needs.

Get Fitted: Ensure the device is adjusted to your height and size.

Practice: Familiarize yourself with the device under your therapist's guidance before solo use.

Beyond Basics: Additional Aids for Independence

Consider these extras to enhance your daily life:

Grab Bars: Install for support in crucial areas like bathrooms.

Reacher's: Handy for grabbing items out of reach.

Sock and Shoe Aids: Make dressing easier.

Shower Chairs and Bath Seats: For safer bathing.

Transfer Benches: Assist with transferring between surfaces.

Dressing Aids: Help with independent dressing.

Using Your Device Safely: Tips for Security

Here's how to stay safe while using your device:

Follow Instructions: Heed guidance from your therapist on device use.

Regular Inspections: Check for damage or wear regularly.

Posture Matters: Maintain good posture to prevent discomfort.

Stay Alert: Be aware of your surroundings, especially in challenging environments.

Ask for Help: Don't hesitate to seek assistance when needed.

Embracing Independence with Assistive Devices

These tools aren't signs of weakness but pathways to independence:

Empowering Tools: Assistive devices help you regain autonomy and enhance your quality of life.

With the Right Device: Proper training and a positive mindset, you can tackle daily activities confidently and safely.

CHAPTER FIVE

REBUILDING COMMUNICATION SKILLS

5.1 SPEECH THERAPY TECHNIQUES FOR APHASIA

Dealing with aphasia post-stroke can be incredibly challenging, but there's light at the end of the tunnel. Speech therapy offers a diverse toolkit to help you regain your voice and reconnect with the world. Let's delve into some effective speech therapy techniques for aphasia, shedding light on how they can empower you in your journey towards effective communication.

Grasping Aphasia: Understanding the Communication Spectrum

Aphasia doesn't follow a one-size-fits-all pattern. Here's a breakdown of its types and the communication hurdles they pose:

1. Expressive Aphasia: Struggle to find the right words.

2. Receptive Aphasia: Difficulty understanding spoken language.

3.Anomic Aphasia: Trouble recalling specific words.

4. Global Aphasia: Severe communication impairment affecting all aspects.

Your Guide on the Path to Recovery: The Speech-Language Pathologist

A speech-language pathologist (SLP) is your ally in this journey. They'll assess your aphasia type and severity and craft a tailored therapy plan. Here's what to expect:

Thorough Evaluation: Assessing your communication skills comprehensively.

Goal Setting: Collaborating with you to set realistic recovery goals.

Therapeutic Techniques: Introducing diverse methods based on your specific aphasia and goals.

Let's explore some common techniques employed in speech therapy for aphasia:

1. Picture Communication: Utilizing images and symbols for nonverbal expression.

2. Melodic Intonation Therapy (MIT): Employing sing-song patterns to enhance speech fluency.

3. Constraint-Induced Aphasia Therapy (CIAT): Maximizing communication opportunities by reducing reliance on alternative methods.

4. Repetition Therapy: Strengthening neural pathways through word repetition.

5. Semantic Feature Analysis: Breaking down word meanings to aid word retrieval.

6. Context Therapy: Providing context clues for better language comprehension.

7. Pragmatic Therapy: Enhancing language use in social contexts.

Nurturing Communication Beyond Therapy Sessions

Speech therapy extends beyond clinical settings. Here's how to bolster communication at home:

Consistent Practice: Integrate communication exercises into daily routines.

Patience: Acknowledge small wins and don't be disheartened by setbacks.

Family Involvement: Educate loved ones on aphasia and encourage their support.

Alternative Methods: Explore aids like picture boards or communication apps.

Support Groups: Connect with others facing similar challenges for mutual encouragement.

Embracing Technology: Harnessing Tools for Communication

Technology offers invaluable support for aphasia:

Speech-generating devices: Transform typed words into synthesized speech.

Communication apps: Provide symbol systems and text-to-speech features.

Augmentative and alternative communication (AAC) devices: Aid those with severe communication difficulties.

The Journey to Recovery: Cultivating Positivity and Support

Recovery from aphasia is a marathon. Here are additional tips to foster a positive, supportive environment:

Positive Outlook: Focus on progress and maintain belief in your ability to communicate effectively.

Celebration: Acknowledge achievements to stay motivated.

Stress Management: Practice relaxation techniques to reduce stress.

Enjoyable Activities: Engage in activities you love for practice.

Support Networks: Connect with fellow survivors for encouragement and advice.

Rediscovering the Joy of Communication

Regaining effective communication post-stroke is empowering. With speech therapy, dedication, and support, you can overcome aphasia's challenges and reconnect with the world. In our next chapter, we'll explore the vital role of nutrition in stroke recovery, offering tips for a heart-healthy diet plan. By integrating effective communication strategies, a balanced diet, and a supportive environment, you can pave the way for a fulfilling life after stroke.

5.2 Strategies for Effective Communication with Others

Dealing with aphasia post-stroke can be a real communication hurdle, affecting your ability to connect with loved ones and navigate social situations smoothly. But here's the bright side: with some adjustments and a bit of teamwork, you can bridge these gaps and foster meaningful communication. Let's dive into strategies for both you and your conversation partners to ensure effective communication post-aphasia.

Understanding Your Communication Style: Identifying Your Strengths

Your communication style may have shifted after a stroke. Here's how to recognize your current strengths and weaknesses:

Self-Assessment: Reflect on what communication methods work best for you—speaking, writing, gestures, or using pictures.

Talk to Your Therapist: Your speech-language pathologist (SLP) can evaluate your communication skills and offer valuable insights.

Effective Communication Strategies for You:

Here are some strategies you can employ to help others understand you better:

Start Simple: Kick off conversations with short, simple sentences, focusing on the main idea.

Use Gestures and Facial Expressions: Nonverbal cues can amplify your message, so utilize gestures, facial expressions, and body language.

Point to Objects or Pictures: When words fail, pointing to objects or pictures can convey your needs more clearly.

Write it Down: If speaking proves challenging, jot down what you want to say, especially in crucial situations like medical appointments.

Speak Slowly and Clearly: Enunciate your words and maintain a steady pace to aid comprehension.

Be Patient: Don't be disheartened if communication takes longer—patience is key for both you and your conversation partner.

Creating a Supportive Communication Environment:

Here are some tips for your conversation partner to ensure smooth interaction:

Be Patient and Attentive: Allow ample time for processing and responding, practicing active listening with eye contact and avoiding interruptions.

Speak Simply and Clearly: Use straightforward language and avoid complexity, speaking at a moderate pace.

Ask Open-Ended Questions: Foster elaborate responses by steering clear of yes or no queries.

Focus on Nonverbal Cues: Pay attention to gestures and expressions for deeper understanding.

Offer Choices: Help by suggesting simple options if finding the right word is a struggle.

Minimize Distractions: Find a quiet space with minimal background noise to aid clear communication.

Be Positive and Encouraging: Celebrate communication successes, no matter how small, to boost confidence and motivation.

Tools and Technology to Bridge the Gap:

Technology can be a game-changer in overcoming communication barriers. Here are some examples:

Speech-generating devices: Transform typed words into synthesized speech.

Communication apps: Offer picture boards, symbol systems, and text-to-speech features.

Augmentative and alternative communication (AAC) devices: Designed for those with severe communication difficulties.

The Power of Collaboration: Working Together for Success

Effective communication post-aphasia is a joint effort. Here's how you and your conversation partner can team up:

Communicate Your Needs: Share your preferred communication methods and any specific challenges with your partner.

Be Patient with Each Other: Understand that recovery takes time and there may be hiccups along the way.

Practice Makes Progress: Keep those communication skills sharp by engaging in conversations with friends, family, and support groups.

Celebrate Milestones: Acknowledge and celebrate every success, big or small, to stay motivated and engaged.

Aphasia doesn't define you. With the right strategies, a positive mindset, and the support of loved ones, you can overcome communication barriers and rebuild meaningful connections with the world around you.

5.3 Tools and Technologies to Aid Communication

Dealing with aphasia can indeed pose communication challenges, but there's a treasure trove of tools and technologies out there ready to help you bridge that gap and express yourself effectively. Let's take a closer look at a range of communication aids, both low-tech and high-tech, tailored to support individuals dealing with aphasia in various ways.

Understanding Your Needs: Selecting the Right Tools

Choosing the right communication aids hinges on your specific needs and the severity of your aphasia. Here are some key points to consider:

1. Type of Aphasia: Different types of aphasia come with their own communication hurdles, so understanding your specific type can guide your tool selection.

2. Communication Strengths and Weaknesses: Knowing where you shine and where you struggle—whether it's speaking, understanding, reading, or writing—can point you towards aids that complement your strongest communication methods.

3. Level of Tech Comfort: If you're not tech-savvy, simpler tools might be less frustrating to navigate.

Low-Tech Communication Aids: Simple Solutions for Daily Needs

Low-tech aids are often affordable and easy to access. Here's a rundown:

Picture Communication Boards: These boards feature images or symbols representing common words, phrases, and activities, offering a straightforward way to convey your needs visually.

Communication Notebooks: Keep a notebook handy with frequently used words and phrases written down for easy reference.

Calendars and Schedules: Visual schedules with pictures or symbols can help you stay organized throughout the day.

Whiteboards and Markers: Ideal for quick jotting down of thoughts or ideas, especially in situations where writing things down is helpful.

Exploring High-Tech Communication Aids: Harnessing the Power of Tech

Technology opens up a world of sophisticated aids for aphasia. Here are some notable examples:

Speech-Generating Devices (SGDs): These electronic devices let you type words or phrases that are then converted into synthesized speech, offering various sizes and functionalities to suit your needs.

Augmentative and Alternative Communication (AAC) Apps: Many mobile apps provide features like picture boards and text-to-speech functionality, offering a portable communication solution.

Communication Software: Computer programs offer word prediction, text-to-speech conversion, and on-screen keyboards to aid written communication.

Eye-Gaze Technology: Advanced tech that enables individuals with limited mobility to control a computer cursor or communication software using eye movements.

Choosing the Right Technology: Finding Help and Support

Navigating the tech landscape can be daunting, but you're not alone. Here's where to turn for guidance:

Speech-Language Pathologist (SLP): Your SLP can assess your needs and recommend suitable communication aids.

Assistive Technology Specialists: These pros can guide you through different technologies, offer training, and customize settings for optimal use.

Aphasia Support Groups: Connecting with others facing similar challenges can provide valuable insights and recommendations.

Learning and Adapting: Mastering Your Tools

Adapting to new communication tools takes time. Here's how to ease into it:

Start Simple: Begin with basic tools or features before moving on to more complex options.

Get Training: Proper training ensures you make the most of your aids.

Practice Regularly: The more you practice, the more comfortable you'll get.

Be Patient: Learning takes time, so be kind to yourself and celebrate progress, no matter how small.

The Future of Communication Technology: Constant Innovation

Assistive technology keeps evolving. Here's a glimpse into what's on the veiw:

Voice Recognition Technology: Improved software could make controlling aids easier through spoken commands.

Brain-Computer Interfaces (BCIs): This emerging tech may translate brain activity into communication outputs, offering new possibilities for those with severe communication challenges.

Communication is a journey, not a Destination

Remember, mastering communication post-aphasia is a journey, not a quick fix. By embracing a mix of low-tech and high-tech aids, coupled with effective strategies, you can conquer hurdles and express yourself with confidence. Stay tuned for the next chapter, where we'll dive into the importance of a healthy diet post-stroke, setting you on a path to recovery and a fulfilling life.

CHAPTER SIX

MANAGING COGNITIVE CHALLENGES

6.1 UNDERSTANDING MEMORY LOSS AND ATTENTION DIFFICULTIES

Experiencing a stroke can throw a wrench into the intricate workings of your brain, affecting vital cognitive functions like memory and attention. While grappling with these hurdles might feel daunting, grasping the reasons behind them and adopting effective strategies can arm you with the tools needed to navigate them and boost your overall well-being.

Unpacking the Impact of Stroke on the Brain

Your brain serves as the command center for your body, orchestrating everything from basic movements to complex thoughts and recollections. When a stroke strikes, it disrupts this flow by impeding blood flow to a portion of the brain, leading to cell death in that region. Depending on where and how severe the stroke is, different cognitive functions can take a hit.

Memory and Attention: Stepping into the Limelight

Two key cognitive functions, memory, and attention, often find themselves squarely in the crosshairs of stroke. Let's zoom in on their roles:

Memory: It involves encoding, storing, and retrieving information, and stroke can throw wrenches into different memory aspects such as:

1. Short-term memory: Struggles to recall recently learned or heard information.

2. Long-term memory: Difficulties in retrieving past events or data.

3. Working memory: Challenges in holding and manipulating information mentally for tasks like following instructions or performing calculations.

Attention: It's about focusing on specific information while filtering out distractions, and stroke can result in:

1. Difficulty concentrating: Trouble sustaining focus on tasks or conversations.

2. Distractibility: Easy diversion of attention by background noise or environmental stimuli.

3. Mental fatigue: Tiring out mentally after prolonged concentration.

Navigating the Spectrum of Memory and Attention Challenges

The severity of memory and attention issues post-stroke varies widely. Here's a spectrum of common experiences:

Mild Impairment: Occasional forgetfulness or time mismanagement but manageable daily activities.

Moderate Impairment: Disruptive memory or attention issues that warrant help with tasks like managing finances or sticking to medication schedules.

Severe Impairment: Major memory or attention problems calling for constant supervision or specialized care.

Pinpointing Your Unique Challenges

The first step toward tackling memory and attention hurdles is recognizing them. Keep an eye out for signs like:

Frequently missed appointments or meds.

Struggles with following conversations or instructions.

Misplacing belongings or losing track of time often.

Difficulty concentrating on tasks or activities.

Increased reliance on memory aids like reminders or notes.

If you suspect memory or attention troubles post-stroke, it's wise to consult your doctor or a neuropsychologist for a thorough evaluation. This can shed light on the specific memory and attention types affected and gauge their severity.

Remember: It's Not Weakness, It's Injury

Memory and attention issues post-stroke aren't a reflection of weakness but rather a consequence of brain injury, manageable with the right strategies and support.

Up Next: Practical Strategies for Coping

In the next section, we'll dive into practical strategies to help you tackle memory and attention challenges post-stroke. By weaving these techniques into your daily routine, you can sharpen your cognitive prowess and reclaim control over your everyday life.

6.2 Strategies for Cognitive Rehabilitation

Experiencing a stroke can throw a wrench into the intricate workings of your brain, affecting memory and attention in ways that can be quite frustrating. But here's the silver lining: cognitive rehabilitation steps in as a specialized therapy approach, empowering you to take back control and boost your cognitive function. Let's dive into the various strategies used in cognitive rehabilitation to tackle memory and attention challenges post-stroke.

Unpacking the Magic of Cognitive Rehabilitation

Cognitive rehabilitation zeroes in on retraining the brain to compensate for areas affected by the stroke. Here's how it works:

Strengthening Existing Pathways: Through repetitive cognitive exercises, you can bolster existing neural pathways, making them more efficient.

Forming New Connections: Harnessing the brain's remarkable plasticity, this therapy encourages the creation of new neural pathways to fill in for damaged ones, thereby boosting cognitive function.

Developing Coping Strategies: Therapists equip you with practical strategies to navigate memory and attention hurdles, making everyday tasks more manageable.

Memory Makeover: Strategies to Remember

When it comes to memory enhancement, cognitive rehabilitation pulls out all the stops with techniques such as:

Repetition and Spaced Practice: Repeating info over time with spaced intervals helps cement memories and improves recall.

Mnemonics: Crafting memory aids like acronyms, rhymes, or vivid imagery can amp up information retention.

Organization Tactics: Setting up organizational systems for tasks, appointments, and belongings reduces memory reliance and amps up overall efficiency.

External Memory Tools: Leveraging tools like calendars, planners, or reminder apps can jog your memory and keep you on track throughout the day.

Visualization: Mental imagery can boost memory encoding and retrieval, especially handy for recalling sequences or directions.

Attention Please: Tips for Sharpening Focus

To combat attention wobbles, cognitive rehabilitation dishes out techniques like:

Attention Training Drills: Engaging in focused activities trains your brain to filter out distractions and maintain attention.

Distraction Detox: Crafting a serene, clutter-free environment amps up your ability to concentrate.

Task Chunking: Breaking down complex tasks into bite-sized chunks amps up focus and task completion efficiency.

Monotasking Mastery: Focusing on one task at a time minimizes divided attention and cuts down on errors.

Take a Breather: Scheduling regular breaks during tasks needing sustained attention helps stave off mental fatigue and keeps focus intact.

Occupational Therapy: The Unsung Hero

Occupational therapists (OTs) swoop in to play a vital role in cognitive rehabilitation by:

Assessing Your Needs: OTs conduct thorough evaluations to pinpoint your specific memory and attention hurdles.

Crafting a Personalized Plan: Armed with insights, they concoct a tailored therapy plan chock-full of evidence-based strategies to tackle your unique challenges.

Practice and Encouragement: Offering ample practice sessions and positive reinforcement, they help you master new cognitive skills.

Educating Caregivers: OTs enlighten your family and caregivers about effective support strategies for your memory and attention challenges in daily life.

Tech to the Rescue: Innovative Tools for Cognitive Rehab

Harnessing the power of technology, cognitive rehabilitation brings forth:

Computerized Training Programs: Interactive software dishes out targeted exercises to buff up memory, attention, and other cognitive skills.

Handy Apps: Mobile apps dish out memory games, organizational tools, and reminders, jazzing up cognitive function in a fun and handy way.

Virtual Reality (VR): Emerging VR tech offers immersive environments for cognitive training and rehabilitation, opening up new avenues for recovery.

Cognitive rehabilitation is no quick fix; it's a gradual journey. Consistent effort, a dollop of patience, and a positive attitude are your trusty companions on this voyage.

Here are some bonus tips to keep you on track:

Embrace a Healthy Lifestyle: A balanced diet, regular exercise, and ample shut-eye are your brain's best buddies.

Tame Stress: Chronic stress can throw a wrench into cognitive function. Unwind with deep breathing exercises or meditation to keep stress at bay.

Stay Engaged: Keep those mental gears oiled by diving into activities like reading, puzzles, or brain teasers.

Celebrate Wins: Every little victory counts, so pat yourself on the back and keep that motivation high.

Navigating the Road to Recovery: A Supportive Ecosystem

Cognitive rehab thrives in a nurturing environment. Here's how your loved ones can lend a helping hand:

Patience and Compassion: Memory and attention stumbles can test everyone's patience. Approach slip-ups with understanding and kindness.

Cueing Up: Gentle reminders or cues can be a lifeline in memory retrieval. Help with appointments, finding lost items, or repeating instructions can make a world of difference.

Chunking Tasks: Breaking down complex tasks into bite-sized chunks makes them more digestible, helping boost focus and reduce frustration.

Routine is Key: A predictable routine adds a comforting rhythm to life, easing memory and attention struggles.

Pep Talks: Showering praise and acknowledging improvements, no matter how small, serves as powerful fuel for the rehab journey.

The Silver Lining: Living Life to the Fullest

Memory and attention hiccups post-stroke needn't put a damper on your life's vibrancy. By embracing cognitive rehabilitation strategies, fostering a healthy lifestyle, and rallying support from loved ones, you can reclaim control, sharpen your cognitive prowess, and bask in newfound independence and well-being.

6.3 Tools and Techniques to Enhance Focus and Memory

Dealing with memory and attention challenges post-stroke can be quite the hurdle, impacting your daily activities and overall well-being. But hey, chin up! There's a plethora of tools and techniques out there waiting to be embraced, helping you sharpen those cognitive skills and reclaim a sense of control.

Understanding Your Cognitive Style: Picking Your Arsenal

When it comes to beefing up focus and memory, the key lies in choosing tools that sync with your individual needs and learning style. Here's the lowdown:

Self-Assessment: Take a moment to figure out how you learn best. Are you a visual learner, someone who thrives on auditory cues, or perhaps you're a fan of jotting things down?

Therapist Chat: Your occupational therapist (OT) is your go-to guru here. They can pinpoint your specific cognitive challenges and hook you up with tools and techniques tailor-made for you.

Try and Tweak: Don't hesitate to dabble in different tools to find your groove. Stay flexible and tweak existing techniques to fit snugly with your learning style and preferences.

Everyday Cognitive Support: Low-Tech Heroes

Low-tech tools are the unsung heroes of your daily grind, easily slotting into your routine. Here are some gems:

Notebooks and Planners: Carrying around a trusty notebook or planner can be a lifesaver for jotting down crucial info, schedules, or reminders.

Calendars and Whiteboards: Visual aids like calendars and whiteboards help keep you on track. Map out your week, prioritize tasks, or drop visual cues for yourself.

Color Coding: Injecting some color into your planner or calendar can jazz up visual recall and make finding specific info a breeze.

Sticky Notes: These little marvels are perfect for quick reminders or flagging important details for later attention.

Timers and Alarms: Set 'em up to nudge you about tasks, appointments, or medication times, especially handy if time management's not your strong suit.

Tech-Powered Focus and Memory Boosts

Technology's a treasure trove of tools to supercharge your cognitive game. Check these out:

Brain-Training Programs: Interactive software dishes out targeted exercises to beef up memory, attention, and more, all while tracking your progress.

Handy Apps: Mobile apps are chock-full of memory games, organizational tools, reminders, and brain-training exercises, all conveniently tucked into your pocket.

Digital Planners: Say hello to digital calendars and planner apps, armed with nifty features like notifications, reminders, and task management tools to keep you on top of things.

Voice Recorders: Capture important deets during lectures, meetings, or chats, then play 'em back later to cement those memories.

Sharpening Your Cognitive Arsenal: Daily Drills

Here are some tried-and-tested strategies to hone your focus and memory:

Mnemonics: Cook up memory aids like acronyms, rhymes, or vivid imagery to turbocharge information retention.

Chunking: Slice and dice vast chunks of info into bite-sized pieces for easier processing and recall.

Active Learning: Dive into info headfirst by taking notes, summarizing key points, or chewing over details with a pal.

Visualization: Paint a mental picture of the info you're grappling with for a little extra oomph.

Practice, Practice, Practice: The more you flex those cognitive muscles, the stronger they'll get. Make these techniques part of your daily grind.

Crafting Your Optimal Learning Nook: The Supportive Environment

The space you inhabit can make or break your focus and memory. Here's how to craft a conducive learning environment:

Organize Your Lair: Whip your workspace into shape, keeping everything, you need within arm's reach to minimize distractions and wasted mental energy.

Break Time: Pencil in regular breaks to stave off brain fatigue. Get up, stretch, or bust out a mini dance party to reboot your focus.

Goals Galore: Don't bite off more than you can chew. Set small, achievable goals, and relish each milestone along the way.

Healthy Habits: Nourish your brain with a balanced diet, regular exercise, and ample shut-eye to keep those cognitive gears turning smoothly.

Enhancing focus and memory post-stroke is a marathon, not a sprint. Be gentle with yourself, cheer on your victories, and lean on your therapist and loved ones when you need a hand. By staying the course with these strategies and picking the right tools, you'll reignite your cognitive prowess and seize the reins of your daily life once more.

CHAPTER SEVEN

NUTRITION FOR STROKE RECOVERY

7.1 FOODS THAT SUPPORT HEALING AND BRAIN HEALTH

After a stroke, your body gears up for a crucial healing phase, and proper nutrition is like fuel for the journey. It not only helps in physical recovery but also boosts your energy levels and supports your brain health. This chapter dives into the vital connection between food and stroke recovery, offering guidance on crafting a diet that's good for your heart and great for your brain.

Understanding the Food-Stroke Recovery Link:

What you eat plays a starring role in your body's healing saga post-stroke. Here's why a healthy diet is your sidekick for recovery:

Essential Nutrients: Your body craves a buffet of vitamins, minerals, proteins, and healthy fats to mend tissues, amp up the immune system, and keep everything ticking.

Inflammation Buster: Certain foods are like superheroes, fighting off inflammation, which can put the brakes on your recovery journey.

Brain Booster: Your noggin gets some special attention post-stroke. Nutrients can help improve blood flow, foster new brain cells, and even amp up your thinking skills.

Blood Pressure and Cholesterol Control: High blood pressure and wonky cholesterol levels often cozy up to strokes. But fear not—a heart-healthy diet can wrangle them into submission and prevent future strokes.

Building a Brain-Boosting Diet Plate:

Now that you're hip to the nutrition scoop, let's dig into some key food groups to load up on after a stroke:

Fruits and Veggies: These colorful gems are chock-full of vitamins, minerals, and antioxidants. Load up your plate with a rainbow of produce for a nutrient-packed feast.

Whole Grains: Fiber is your friend here, helping with digestion and blood sugar control. Opt for the whole grain gang—brown rice, quinoa, oats, and whole-wheat bread.

Lean Protein: Proteins like the building block for repairing tissues and keeping those muscles in tip-top shape. Think fish, chicken, turkey, beans, and legumes.

Healthy Fats: Your brain's BFFs are omega-3s and monounsaturated fats. Show some love with fatty fish, avocados, nuts, seeds, and olive oil.

Low-Fat Dairy: These goodies are bursting with calcium and vitamin D for those bones.

Foods to Nix or Nibble Less:

Watch out for these troublemakers in your diet post-stroke:

- Saturated and Trans Fats: They're the villains that hike up your "bad" cholesterol and put you at risk for heart woes. Keep tabs on fried foods, processed meats, and their cronies.

- Added Sugars: They sneak into drinks, snacks, and treats, setting the stage for weight gain and inflammation. Go easy on the sweet stuff and reach for nature's candy—fruits.

- Sodium: Too much salt's like a red carpet for high blood pressure. Ease up on processed foods, canned goods, and the salt shaker.

A Stroke-Recovery Meal Plan:

Peek at this sample meal plan for some inspo on how to whip up stroke-friendly meals:

Breakfast: Oatmeal with berries and walnuts, a side of low-fat yogurt with banana and chia seeds.

Lunch: Grilled salmon, roasted veggies, and brown rice, plus a fresh salad with vinaigrette.

Dinner: Chicken stir-fry with whole-wheat noodles and veggies, served with a glass of low-fat milk.

Snacks: Fresh fruits with nut butter, veggie sticks with hummus, and air-popped popcorn.

Making Healthy Eating Stick:

Turning over a new leaf with your diet post-stroke takes some TLC. Here's how to make it stick:

Meal Planning: Sketch out your meals and snacks for the week to dodge unhealthy picks when you're pressed for time.

Prep Ahead: Batch-cook meals or snacks in advance to save time and ensure healthier options are always at arm's reach.

Get Cooking: Whip up meals at home to keep tabs on ingredients and portion sizes.

Label Love: Scrutinize food labels for the deets. Keep an eye on sodium, sugar, and sat fat content.

Shop Smart: Load up on whole foods and dial back on processed stuff during your grocery hauls.

Rally the Troops: Rope in friends or fam to help with meal planning, cooking sessions, or just to keep you on track.

Slow and Steady: Rome wasn't built in a day, and neither is a new diet. Ease into changes gradually for long-lasting results.

Treat your Self: Don't forget to indulge every now and then. A little splurge here and there keeps things balanced.

Listen to Your Body: Tune in to how different foods make you feel. Stick with the ones that keep you buzzing with energy and focus.

A healthy diet isn't just a pit stop—it's a roadmap for your stroke recovery journey. By blending these tips and loading up on nutrient-rich foods, you're not just feeding your body; you're nourishing your mind, kickstarting healing, and paving.

7.2 Creating a Healthy Stroke-Friendly Diet

Experiencing a stroke throws quite a curveball, impacting not just your physical health but also your emotional well-being. Nutrition steps up as a crucial player in this recovery game, and this chapter is all about tailoring your diet to suit your unique needs and preferences, ultimately fostering your overall well-being.

Going Beyond the Basics: Customizing Your Diet

While we've covered the fundamentals of a stroke-friendly diet earlier, it's vital to understand that there's no one-size-fits-all solution. Here's how you can tweak your diet plan to match your journey:

Consider Existing Conditions: If you're dealing with diabetes, high blood pressure, or other health conditions, your diet might need some extra tailoring. Team up with a doctor or registered dietitian (RD) to craft a plan that's spot-on for you.

Dietary Restrictions or Allergies: Got any food allergies or dietary restrictions? Ensure your diet plan is a safe zone for you. For instance, if dairy's a no-go, explore calcium-rich alternatives like leafy greens or fortified plant-based milks.

Cultural Roots and Culinary Preferences: Food's not just fuel; it's culture and comfort. Honor your culinary heritage while embracing stroke-friendly picks. Dive into healthy recipes and culinary traditions that resonate with your roots.

Partnering Up with a Registered Dietitian:

An RD can be your wingman in sculpting a diet that's tailor-made for your stroke recovery journey. Here's how they can lend a hand:

Nutritional Checkup: They'll dive into your health history, medical records, and dietary quirks to craft a personalized plan.

Setting Goals: Together, you'll carve out realistic dietary goals that sync up with your recovery pace.

Meal Masterminding: Need some meal prep magic? An RD's got you covered with stroke-friendly recipes, smart meal planning tips, and tasty swaps.

Grocery Guidance: Navigate the aisles like a pro with their expert tips on picking the best fuel for your recovery journey.

Cheers and Support: Think of them as your cheerleader, offering motivation and a listening ear as you navigate the twists and turns of dietary changes.

Beyond the Plate: Life Influences on Your Diet

Your diet dance extends beyond what's on your plate. Here's how lifestyle factors can sway your dietary groove:

Physical Ability: If your stroke's thrown a wrench in your physical prowess, adapt your kitchen setup or seek a helping hand with meal prep to keep things cooking.

Fatigue Management: Fatigue's a real deal after a stroke. Whip up meals that are light on prep and easy on the tummy for those low-energy days.

Social Sizzle: Don't let a stroke dim your social sparkle. Find ways to gather 'round the table with loved ones, even if it means tweaking traditions to suit your new normal.

Crafting a Diet that Sticks:

Creating lasting dietary changes calls for a game plan. Here's how to make your stroke-friendly diet a keeper:

Baby Steps: Rome wasn't built in a day, and neither is a new diet. Ease into changes, savoring each small win along the way.

Keep It Real: Set achievable goals, like adding a new veggie to your plate each week. Celebrate every milestone and gradually level up your goals.

Snack Swap: Crave something crunchy or sweet? Swap out the usual suspects for healthier picks like fruit with a sprinkle of spice or popcorn jazzed up with a dash of herbs.

Cooking Crew: Turn meal prep into a party by roping in pals or family. Get creative in the kitchen together, exploring new flavors and bonding over bites.

Stay Hydrated: Water's your BFF for recovery. Guzzle up those eight glasses a day and load up on hydrating fruits and veggies for an extra boost.

Crafting a diet that's your perfect match takes time and patience. Celebrate every victory, big or small, and lean on your healthcare squad or an RD when you need a boost. With a customized diet plan and a positive mindset, you're paving the way for a thriving stroke recovery journey.

7.3 Managing Weight and Maintaining Good Nutrition

Experiencing a stroke brings significant changes to your body's needs and capabilities. This shift makes maintaining a healthy weight and nourishing your body with good nutrition even more vital for your recovery and long-term health. In this chapter, we'll delve into why managing your weight post-stroke is crucial and offer guidance on how to strike the right balance between healthy eating and weight management.

The Weight-Stroke Connection:

Keeping a healthy weight post-stroke comes with a plethora of perks. Here's why it's so important:

Less Strain on Your Heart: Shedding excess weight eases the burden on your heart, which is already working hard post-stroke. Managing your weight can boost heart health and slash the risk of future issues.

Enhanced Mobility: Maintaining a healthy weight bolsters your mobility and independence, letting you dive back into daily activities more actively.

Combatting Inflammation: Obesity tends to stoke the fires of chronic inflammation, which can impede healing and worsen stroke outcomes.

Sharper Mind: Research hints at a connection between managing weight effectively and improved cognitive function post-stroke.

Weight Changes Post-Stroke:

Post-stroke, your scale might swing in different directions. Here's why:

Activity Levels Take a Hit: Limited movement post-stroke can dial down your calorie burn, potentially nudging the scale upwards.

Swallowing Struggles: Difficulty swallowing can make it tough to hit your calorie quota, leading to weight loss.

Emotional Rollercoaster: The emotional fallout from a stroke might mess with your appetite, nudging your weight in either direction.

Striking the Right Balance:

Navigating weight management post-stroke boils down to finding harmony between healthy eating and maintaining a healthy weight. Here's how:

Load Up on Good Stuff: Pack your plate with whole foods bursting with nutrients, like vitamins, minerals, and fiber. They're not just filling; they're key for healing and overall health.

Mind the Portions: Even the healthiest fare can tip the scales if you go overboard. Tune into mindful eating and watch those portion sizes.

Team Up with the Pros: Chat with your doc or a registered dietitian (RD) about your weight goals. They'll whip up a personalized plan that's got your back, stroke quirks and all.

Calories Count: Your daily calorie needs post-stroke hinge on your activity levels and pre-stroke weight. An RD can help you nail down your magic number to support both weight management and your recovery journey.

Tackling Nutritional Hurdles:

Here are some specific nutrition roadblocks you might encounter post-stroke, along with savvy solutions:

Swallowing Snags (Dysphagia): Speech therapists can arm you with smart swallowing techniques and dish out tips on thickened liquids or pureed goodies to keep your calorie game strong.

Appetite Amnesia: If your appetite's playing hide-and-seek, opt for calorie-dense foods in small servings. Think healthy fats or protein powders jazzing up your smoothies or soups without bulking up the volume.

Fatigue Factor: Whip up meals that are easy-peasy to prepare and won't drain your batteries. Lean on pre-chopped veggies, frozen fruits, or ready-to-go proteins to keep kitchen fatigue at bay.

Embracing a Holistic Lifestyle:

A well-rounded lifestyle that blends diet and exercise is the golden ticket for weight management and overall well-being post-stroke. Here's how to nail it:

Move That Body: Even baby steps count! Dive into activities that suit your groove, be it leisurely strolls, seated workouts, or a splash in the pool.

Stay Hydrated: Guzzle up that H2O to stay full and fend off cravings. Aim for eight glasses daily and toss hydrating fruits and veggies into the mix.

Catch Those Zzz's: Quality sleep's a game-changer, regulating hunger hormones and metabolism. Shoot for 7-8 hours of shut-eye each night.

Chill Out: Stress messes with your eating patterns and weight goals. Tackle it head-on with relaxation hacks like deep breathing or meditation.

Weight management post-stroke is a marathon, not a sprint. Take it slow, celebrate every victory, and lean on your healthcare crew or an RD when the going gets tough. With a dash of patience, a dollop of healthy eating, and a sprinkle of balance, you're well on your way to managing your weight like a boss and paving the road to overall well-being post-stroke.

CHAPTER EIGHT

REGAINING CONTROL OF YOUR HEALTH

8.1 MANAGING BLOOD PRESSURE AND CHOLESTEROL

Experiencing a stroke is like a wake-up call for our heart health. Conditions like high blood pressure and unhealthy cholesterol levels are significant red flags for strokes. Post-stroke, managing these factors becomes even more crucial to steer clear of future complications. In this chapter, we'll dive deep into understanding blood pressure and cholesterol, explore ways to manage them, and highlight the importance of a proactive approach.

Understanding Blood Pressure and Its Impact:

Blood pressure is the force exerted by your blood against artery walls. Here's how it affects your health:

Normal Blood Pressure: A healthy reading is typically below 120/80 mmHg, indicating smooth blood flow throughout your body.

High Blood Pressure (Hypertension): Consistent readings above 140/90 mmHg signal hypertension, stressing your heart and blood vessels and upping the odds of stroke and other cardiovascular issues.

Stroke and Blood Pressure: High blood pressure weakens vessel walls, making them prone to rupture or blockage, which can set off a stroke.

Understanding Cholesterol and Its Role:

Cholesterol is a waxy substance in your blood. While it's necessary for certain functions, too much can spell trouble:

Types of Cholesterol: LDL ("bad") cholesterol clogs arteries, while HDL ("good") cholesterol clears out LDL from your bloodstream.

Stroke and Cholesterol: High LDL and low HDL levels pave the way for plaque buildup, narrowing arteries and heightening stroke risk.

Managing Blood Pressure and Cholesterol After Stroke:

After a stroke, keeping tabs on blood pressure and cholesterol is key to warding off future issues. Here's how to tackle it:

Lifestyle Tweaks: Slimming down, staying active, eating heart-healthy, and stress management are game-changers for both blood pressure and cholesterol. (For more on this, check out Chapters 6.1 and 7.)

Medication: Your doc might prescribe meds like diuretics or statins to rein in blood pressure and cholesterol.

Regular Check-Ins: Schedule routine visits to monitor these levels and fine-tune your treatment plan as needed.

The Importance of a Preventive Approach:

While managing blood pressure and cholesterol post-stroke is vital, prevention steals the show. Here's why:

Slash Stroke Risk: By keeping blood pressure and cholesterol in check, you significantly slash the chances of a repeat stroke.

Boost Overall Health: Maintaining healthy levels benefits your heart health overall, cutting the risk of heart attacks and other complications.

Up Your Quality of Life: Living heart-healthy means more energy and a better quality of life.

Working with Your Healthcare Crew:

Your healthcare squad is your ace in the hole for managing blood pressure and cholesterol post-stroke. Here's how they've got your back:

Customized Game Plan: Your doc will tailor a treatment plan to your needs and history.

Med Management: They'll dish out the right meds and keep an eye on how they're working for you.

Education and Support: Your team will school you on why these matters and guide you on living the heart-healthy life.

It's a Marathon, not a Sprint

Managing blood pressure and cholesterol after a stroke is a long-haul gig. But by teaming up with your healthcare posse, embracing a heart-healthy lifestyle, and sticking to your plan, you're stacking the odds in your favor for a healthier, brighter future.

8.2 Maintaining Diabetes Control if Present

If you're living with diabetes, you know that keeping your blood sugar levels in check is key for your overall well-being. But after experiencing a stroke, managing those levels becomes even more crucial. This chapter dives into the link between diabetes and strokes, offers strategies for effective diabetes management post-stroke, and stresses the importance of teaming up with your healthcare crew.

Understanding the Diabetes-Stroke Connection:

Diabetes significantly heightens the risk of stroke. Here's how:

High Blood Sugar: Chronically elevated blood sugar levels can harm blood vessels, making them prone to narrowing or blockage, potentially leading to a stroke.

Inflammation: Diabetes contributes to ongoing inflammation in the body, which further amps up the risk of stroke.

Other Risk Factors: Diabetes often goes hand-in-hand with other stroke risk factors like high blood pressure and unhealthy cholesterol levels.

The Importance of Tight Glycemic Control After Stroke:

Post-stroke, keeping your blood sugar levels in check is paramount. Here's why:

Reduce Stroke Risk: Nailing down good blood sugar control significantly slashes the odds of another stroke down the line.

Boost Recovery: Keeping those levels stable can speed up healing and improve your overall recovery.

Cut Complications: Uncontrolled diabetes post-stroke can hike up the risk of complications like infections and slow wound healing.

Strategies for Effective Diabetes Management After Stroke:

Juggling diabetes post-stroke calls for a holistic approach. Here's how to tackle it:

Regular Monitoring: Keep tabs on your blood sugar levels to gauge how food, meds, and activity impact them. Your doc can help set up a monitoring routine tailored to you.

Healthy Eating: Load up on balanced, heart-healthy grub—think whole foods, fruits, veggies, and lean proteins. (Check out Chapter 7 for the lowdown on whipping up a stroke-friendly diabetic diet.)

Get Moving: Work some physical activity into your routine, based on what you can handle. Your PT can help craft a safe, effective exercise plan post-stroke.

Medication Tweaks: Your doc might adjust your diabetes meds or add new ones to fine-tune your blood sugar control.

Stay Connected: Keep those lines of communication open with your healthcare squad. Share any hurdles you're facing, talk meds, and voice any concerns you have.

Addressing Additional Challenges:

Post-stroke, you might hit some extra roadblocks in managing your diabetes. Here's how to navigate them:

Physical Limits: If stroke-related mobility issues make exercise and meal prep tough, chat with your healthcare crew about workarounds that fit your situation.

Emotional Strain: Coping with the aftermath of a stroke can throw a wrench in your eating habits and motivation to manage diabetes. Reach out to your doc or a therapist for stress-busting strategies.

Tiredness: Post-stroke fatigue is no joke. Plan your blood sugar checks and meals for when you've got the most energy, and look into time-saving meal prep tricks to sidestep fatigue-related hurdles.

The Power of Teamwork:

Teaming up with your healthcare squad is key for acing diabetes management post-stroke. Here's why it's a game-changer:

Tailored Approach: Your doc will craft a plan that's all about you—factoring in your unique needs, stroke aftermath, and any existing diabetes game plan.

Ongoing Backup: Your crew will be there to cheer you on, track your progress, and tweak your plan as needed.

Feeling Empowered: Working in sync with your team puts you in the driver's seat of your health journey, giving you the tools to take charge and set yourself up for long-term success.

Nailing diabetes management after a stroke takes time and teamwork. By leaning on your healthcare crew, embracing healthy habits, and tackling any bumps in the road head-on, you're paving the way for a healthier, brighter tomorrow post-stroke.

8.3 Quitting Smoking and Reducing Alcohol Consumption

A stroke is a major wake-up call, reminding many to prioritize their health. Smoking and excessive alcohol consumption are significant risk factors for stroke. After a stroke, quitting smoking and reducing alcohol intake are crucial steps towards preventing future complications and promoting overall well-being. This chapter explores the harmful effects of smoking and alcohol on post-stroke health, strategies for quitting smoking and reducing alcohol consumption, and the benefits of a smoke-free, low-alcohol lifestyle.

The Dangers of Smoking After Stroke:

Smoking greatly increases the risk of stroke and worsens health outcomes post-stroke. Here's why quitting is essential:

Damaged Blood Vessels: Smoking harms the lining of blood vessels, making them more prone to narrowing or blockage, which can lead to stroke.

Increased Blood Pressure: Smoking raises blood pressure, putting extra strain on the cardiovascular system and increasing the risk of another stroke.

Reduced Oxygen Supply: Smoking decreases the amount of oxygen carried by red blood cells, hindering oxygen delivery to the brain, which is vital for proper functioning.

The Impact of Alcohol on Post-Stroke Health:

While moderate alcohol consumption might have some health benefits for certain individuals, excessive intake can be harmful after a stroke. Here's how it can affect your recovery:

Interaction with Medications: Alcohol can interfere with medications you might be taking post-stroke, reducing their effectiveness or causing adverse side effects.

Increased Blood Pressure: Excessive drinking can raise blood pressure, a significant risk factor for stroke recurrence.

Impaired Cognitive Function: Alcohol can impair cognitive function, which can hinder your rehabilitation progress after a stroke.

Making the Quit: Strategies for Kicking the Smoking Habit:

Quitting smoking can be challenging, but the benefits for your post-stroke health are undeniable. Here are some strategies to help you succeed:

Set a Quit Date: Choose a specific date to quit smoking and commit to it wholeheartedly.

Identify Triggers: Recognize situations or emotions that make you crave a cigarette. Develop coping mechanisms to manage these triggers without resorting to smoking.

Nicotine Replacement Therapy (NRT): Consider using NRT products like patches, gum, or lozenges to manage withdrawal symptoms and cravings.

Seek Support: Talk to your doctor about a smoking cessation program or join a support group to connect with others who are also quitting.

Focus on the Benefits: Remind yourself of the positive reasons you're quitting—improved health, reduced risk of stroke recurrence, and a longer, healthier life.

Moderation is Key: Strategies for Reducing Alcohol Consumption:

If you drink alcohol, reducing your intake after a stroke is crucial. Here are some tips to help you moderate your drinking:

Set Limits: Establish daily or weekly limits for alcohol consumption and stick to them.

Pace Yourself: If you choose to drink, sip your beverage slowly and alternate alcoholic drinks with water to avoid overconsumption.

Find Alternatives: Explore non-alcoholic beverages you enjoy to socialize without relying on alcohol.

Seek Support: Talk to your doctor about your desire to moderate your alcohol intake. They can offer guidance and support.

Focus on the Benefits: Acknowledge the positive outcomes of reduced alcohol consumption, such as improved blood pressure, better sleep, and enhanced cognitive function.

Reaping the Rewards of a Smoke-Free, Low-Alcohol Lifestyle:

Quitting smoking and reducing alcohol consumption offer numerous benefits after a stroke. Here's what you can expect:

Reduced Risk of Future Strokes: By eliminating smoking and limiting alcohol intake, you significantly decrease your risk of experiencing another stroke.

Improved Overall Health: Quitting smoking and drinking less contribute to better cardiovascular health, improved lung function, and a stronger immune system.

Enhanced Recovery: A smoke-free, low-alcohol lifestyle promotes faster healing, improved cognitive function, and increased energy levels, aiding your stroke recovery journey.

Better Quality of Life: By prioritizing a healthier lifestyle, you can experience a significant improvement in your overall well-being and quality of life.

Remember,

Quitting smoking and reducing alcohol consumption are not easy feats. Don't be discouraged by setbacks. Celebrate your progress, no matter how small, and seek support from your healthcare team, family, and friends. With dedication and the right resources, you can achieve a smoke-free, low-alcohol future, paving the way for a healthier and more fulfilling life after stroke.

CHAPTER NINE

PRIORITIZING SLEEP AND STRESS MANAGEMENT

9.1 CREATING A HEALTHY SLEEP ROUTINE FOR RECOVERY

A good night's sleep is crucial for everyone, and even more so after a stroke. Sleep plays a vital role in physical and mental recovery, promoting healing, enhancing cognitive function, and improving overall well-being. This chapter explores the importance of sleep after a stroke, strategies for creating a healthy sleep routine, and tips for overcoming common sleep problems that can arise post-stroke.

The Power of Sleep After Stroke

While you sleep, your body undergoes a restorative process. Here's how sleep benefits your recovery after a stroke:

Physical Repair: During sleep, your body releases hormones that promote tissue repair and muscle growth, which are crucial for healing.

Cognitive Enhancement: Sleep is essential for memory consolidation and cognitive function. Adequate sleep improves focus, concentration, and learning ability, all vital for stroke rehabilitation.

Emotional Regulation: Sleep deprivation can worsen your emotional state. Adequate sleep helps regulate emotions and promotes emotional well-being, which is important for coping with the challenges of stroke recovery.

Boosted Immunity: Sleep strengthens the immune system, making your body more resilient against infections and illnesses, which can hinder recovery.

Building a Sleep-Supportive Routine

Creating a consistent sleep routine is key to promoting good quality sleep after a stroke. Here are some strategies to establish a healthy sleep pattern:

Set a Regular Sleep Schedule: Go to bed and wake up at the same time each day, even on weekends. This helps regulate your body's natural sleep-wake cycle (circadian rhythm).

Create a Relaxing Bedtime Routine: Develop a calming pre-bed routine that signals to your body it's time to wind down. This could include taking a warm bath, reading a book, or listening to soothing music.

Optimize Your Sleep Environment: Ensure your bedroom is dark, quiet, cool, and clutter-free. Invest in blackout curtains, earplugs, and a comfortable mattress and pillows to create an environment conducive to sleep.

Limit Screen Time Before Bed: The blue light emitted from electronic devices can interfere with sleep. Avoid using electronic devices for at least an hour before bedtime.

Regular Exercise: Engage in regular physical activity, but avoid strenuous workouts close to bedtime. Exercise promotes better sleep quality, but vigorous activity should be avoided within three hours of sleep.

Develop a Relaxing Wind-Down Routine: Include calming activities before bedtime, such as light stretching, deep breathing exercises, or meditation. This helps ease anxieties and prepare your mind for sleep.

Addressing Common Sleep Problems After Stroke

Following a stroke, you might experience sleep disturbances such as insomnia, sleep apnea, or fragmented sleep. Here's how to address these common challenges:

1. Insomnia: If you have difficulty falling asleep or staying asleep, avoid napping during the day. Practice relaxation techniques before bed and limit caffeine and alcohol intake, especially in the afternoon and evening.

2. Sleep Apnea: Sleep apnea is a condition where breathing repeatedly stops and starts during sleep. If you suspect sleep apnea, consult your doctor for a diagnosis and treatment plan, which might include using a CPAP (continuous positive airway pressure) machine.

3. Fragmented Sleep: Certain medications or pain after a stroke can disrupt sleep continuity. Discuss these issues with your doctor to explore alternative medications or pain management strategies.

Note that,

Good sleep is essential for your recovery after a stroke. By establishing a consistent sleep routine and addressing any sleep disturbances, you can enhance your physical healing, cognitive function, and overall well-being. Prioritize sleep as a vital part of your recovery journey.

9.2 Relaxation Techniques for Stress Management

A stroke can be a life-altering event, leaving you dealing with physical limitations, emotional challenges, and uncertainty about the future. Stress is a natural response to these difficulties, but chronic stress can hinder your recovery and overall well-being. This chapter explores the impact of stress after a stroke, introduces various relaxation techniques, and empowers you to manage stress effectively and promote emotional health.

The Impact of Stress After Stroke

Stress triggers your body's fight-or-flight response. While short-term stress can be beneficial, chronic stress after a stroke can have negative effects:

Hinders Recovery: Stress hormones like cortisol can impede the tissue repair and healing processes crucial for stroke recovery.

Exacerbates Physical Symptoms: Stress can worsen spasticity, pain, and fatigue, which are common after a stroke.

Contributes to Emotional Distress: Chronic stress can increase anxiety, depression, and feelings of isolation, impacting your emotional well-being.

The Power of Relaxation

Learning relaxation techniques is a powerful tool for managing stress after a stroke. These techniques help activate your body's relaxation response, counteracting the negative effects of stress and promoting emotional well-being. Here's how relaxation can help:

Reduces Stress Hormones: Relaxation techniques lower cortisol levels, promoting healing and reducing the negative physical effects of stress.

Improves Sleep Quality: By calming your mind and body, relaxation techniques can enhance sleep quality, which is essential for overall recovery.

Enhances Emotional Well-Being: Relaxation techniques can alleviate anxiety, depression, and feelings of being overwhelmed, promoting emotional balance and resilience.

Exploring Relaxation Techniques

There's no one-size-fits-all approach to relaxation. Experiment and find techniques that resonate with you. Here are some popular options to explore:

Deep Breathing Exercises: Focused, slow, and deep breathing activates the relaxation response. Techniques like diaphragmatic breathing, where you breathe deeply from your abdomen, can be very effective.

Progressive Muscle Relaxation: This technique involves tensing and then relaxing different muscle groups, bringing awareness to bodily tension and releasing it.

Guided Imagery: Close your eyes and visualize calming scenes or experiences. Imagine yourself on a peaceful beach, surrounded by nature, or in a safe and tranquil environment.

Mindfulness Meditation: Focus your attention on the present moment without judgment. Observe your thoughts and feelings without getting caught up in them. Mindfulness apps can be a helpful resource for beginners.

Relaxation Through Movement: Gentle yoga postures, tai chi, or mindful walking can promote relaxation and improve physical well-being.

Finding What Works for You

The key to successful stress management is finding relaxation techniques that you enjoy and can incorporate into your daily routine. Here are some tips to help you:

Start Small: Begin with short practice sessions and gradually increase the duration as you become more comfortable.

Practice Regularly: The benefits of relaxation techniques accumulate over time. Aim for daily practice, even if it's just for a few minutes.

Create a Relaxing Environment: Find a quiet and comfortable space free from distractions where you can fully focus on relaxation.

Be Patient: Learning relaxation techniques takes practice. Don't get discouraged if you don't experience immediate results.

Combine Techniques: Experiment with different techniques and find combinations that work best for you.

Managing stress after a stroke is crucial for your recovery and overall well-being. By incorporating relaxation techniques into your daily routine, you can reduce stress, improve your physical and emotional health, and enhance your quality of life. Take the time to explore different methods and find what works best for you. With patience and practice, you can make a positive impact on your recovery journey.

9.3 The Importance of Mindfulness and Meditation

Following a stroke, life can feel uncertain and overwhelming. Mindfulness and meditation offer powerful tools to navigate this new reality. These practices cultivate present-moment awareness, helping you manage stress, cope with emotional challenges, and find inner peace during your recovery journey. This chapter explores the benefits of mindfulness and meditation after a stroke, delves into different practices, and provides guidance for incorporating them into your daily routine.

The Power of Mindfulness

Mindfulness is the practice of paying attention to the present moment without judgment. It involves focusing on your thoughts, feelings, and bodily sensations with an attitude of curiosity and acceptance. Here's how mindfulness can benefit you after a stroke:

Reduces Stress and Anxiety: By anchoring your attention to the present, mindfulness helps you detach from worries about the future or regrets about the past, reducing stress and anxiety.

Improves Emotional Regulation: Mindfulness helps you observe your emotions without judgment and develop healthy coping mechanisms for managing them.

Enhances Focus and Concentration: A stroke can impact your attention span. Mindfulness practices can improve focus and concentration, aiding in rehabilitation and daily activities.

Promotes Acceptance: Coming to terms with the limitations and changes after a stroke can be challenging. Mindfulness fosters acceptance of your current situation, allowing you to move forward with greater peace.

Meditation: A Gateway to Mindfulness

Meditation is a form of mindfulness practice that involves focusing your attention on a specific object, thought, or sensation. Here's how meditation can support your recovery:

Reduces Pain Perception: Mindfulness meditation can help you manage chronic pain, a common symptom after a stroke, by shifting your focus away from the pain sensation.

Improves Sleep Quality: Meditation promotes relaxation and reduces stress hormones, contributing to better sleep quality, which is crucial for healing and cognitive function.

Boosts Self-Compassion: Through mindfulness practices, you cultivate kindness and understanding towards yourself, fostering self-compassion during a challenging time.

Exploring Different Meditation Techniques

There are various meditation techniques, each with its own approach. Here are a few popular options to explore:

Focused Attention Meditation: Focus your attention on a single point, such as your breath, a mantra (a repeated word or phrase), or a candle flame. Whenever your mind wanders, gently bring your attention back to the chosen focus.

Body Scan Meditation: Focus your awareness on different parts of your body, noticing any sensations without judgment. This can help you identify and release tension held in your muscles.

Loving-Kindness Meditation: Cultivate feelings of goodwill and compassion towards yourself and others. By focusing on positive affirmations, you can foster self-love and acceptance.

Guided Meditation: Use recordings with verbal instructions to lead you through a specific practice. These can be a helpful resource for beginners.

Finding Your Meditation Practice

The most effective meditation technique is the one that resonates with you and fits your needs. Here are some tips to get started:

Start Small: Begin with short meditation sessions (5-10 minutes) and gradually increase the duration as you become more comfortable.

Find a Quiet Place: Choose a quiet, distraction-free space where you can relax and focus on your practice.

Sit Comfortably: Sit in a comfortable position, either upright in a chair or on the floor with your back supported.

Be Patient: Learning meditation takes practice. Don't get discouraged if your mind wanders. Gently redirect your focus back to your chosen meditation anchor.

Join a Meditation Class: Consider joining a local meditation class or group to learn different techniques and receive support from others.

Mindfulness and meditation are not about achieving a state of perfect calmness or clearing your mind of all thoughts. They're about cultivating present-moment awareness and learning to observe your thoughts and feelings without judgment. By incorporating these practices into your daily routine, you can find inner peace, manage stress more effectively, and navigate the emotional challenges that arise after a stroke.

CHAPTER TEN

REDEFINING YOUR ROLE AND PURPOSE

10.1 EXPLORING NEW ACTIVITIES AND INTERESTS

A stroke can significantly disrupt your life, impacting your physical abilities and daily routines. While it's essential to navigate these changes, it's equally important to embrace new opportunities for growth and rediscover your zest for life. This chapter explores the importance of exploring new activities and interests after a stroke, provides strategies for finding new passions, and offers encouragement for embracing a fulfilling and engaging life.

Rediscovering Yourself After a Stroke

After a stroke, you might find yourself questioning and redefining your identity. Activities you once enjoyed may no longer be feasible in the same way. However, this can also be an opportunity to explore new avenues and discover hidden passions. Here's why embracing new activities and interests is vital after a stroke:

Combating Boredom and Frustration: Focusing on new possibilities can help replace feelings of boredom and frustration that arise from limitations.

Promoting Well-Being: Engaging in activities you enjoy provides a sense of purpose and accomplishment, boosting your overall well-being.

Enhancing Socialization: Exploring new activities can connect you with others who share similar interests, fostering social connections and combating feelings of isolation.

Discovering Hidden Talents: A stroke might necessitate adaptations, but it can also open doors to discovering new talents and abilities you never knew you had.

Finding Your Spark: Strategies for Exploring New Activities

Unsure where to start? Here are some strategies to spark your exploration of new activities and interests:

Reflect on Your Values: Consider what brings you joy and fulfillment. Do you value creativity, physical activity, social interaction, or intellectual stimulation? Let these values guide your exploration.

Revisit Past Passions: Think about activities you enjoyed before your stroke. Can you adapt these activities or find similar alternatives that fit your current abilities?

Explore Your Surroundings: Check your local community center, senior center, or online resources for classes, clubs, or events that pique your interest.

Talk to Others: Seek inspiration from friends, family, or stroke support groups. Explore activities they enjoy and see if anything resonates with you.

Embrace New Challenges: Don't be afraid to step outside your comfort zone. Try something completely new—you might discover a hidden talent you never knew existed.

Adapting Activities and Embracing Modifications

Remember, limitations don't have to define your possibilities. Here are some tips for adapting activities to suit your needs:

Focus on Ability, Not Disability: Shift your mindset. Consider what activities you can do, rather than what you can't.

Seek Assistive Technology: Explore assistive devices or technology that can help you participate in activities you enjoy. Talk to your occupational therapist for recommendations.

Modify Activities: Many activities can be modified to accommodate physical limitations. For instance, you might try seated yoga instead of traditional yoga poses.

Start Small and Build Up: Don't try to do too much too soon. Begin with shorter sessions and gradually increase the duration and intensity as your stamina and skills improve.

Celebrate Your Achievements: Acknowledge and celebrate your progress, no matter how small. Every step forward is a victory!

By exploring new activities and interests, you can find joy and fulfillment in ways you might not have imagined. Embrace this opportunity to rediscover yourself, adapt to new challenges, and live a rich and engaging life after your stroke.

10.2 Adapting Existing Hobbies and Passions

A stroke can disrupt your daily routine and the activities that once brought you joy. Whether it's gardening, photography, playing music, or woodworking, limitations after a stroke might make it seem like you can no longer enjoy these cherished hobbies. However, with a bit of creativity and adaptation, you can reignite your passions and rediscover the joy in your favorite activities. This chapter explores strategies for adapting existing hobbies after a stroke, offers tips for overcoming challenges, and emphasizes the importance of maintaining activities that bring you fulfillment.

The Importance of Existing Hobbies After a Stroke

Continuing to engage in the activities you love offers numerous benefits during your recovery. Here's why adapting your hobbies is crucial:

Preserves Identity: Participating in familiar activities helps you maintain a sense of self and connect with who you were before the stroke.

Promotes Cognitive Function: Many hobbies stimulate cognitive skills like memory, problem-solving, and focus, which can benefit your cognitive recovery.

Improves Mood and Well-Being: Engaging in activities you enjoy reduces stress, promotes feelings of accomplishment, and boosts overall well-being.

Maintains Social Connection: Hobbies can connect you with others who share similar interests, fostering social interaction and combating isolation.

Adapting Your Favorite Activities

While adjustments might be necessary, don't give up on the activities you love. Here are some strategies to adapt your hobbies and continue your passions after a stroke:

Focus on Ability: Shift your mindset from what you can't do to what you can do. Identify aspects of your hobbies you can still participate in and explore ways to modify the activity.

Break Down Tasks: Large tasks can feel overwhelming. Break down your hobbies into smaller, more manageable steps. This makes them more achievable and less daunting.

Seek Assistive Technology: Many assistive devices and technologies can help you continue your hobbies. Explore options like ergonomic tools, voice-activated software, or specialized equipment.

Modify Your Approach: Think outside the box! Can you use different tools, techniques, or approaches to achieve the same outcome? For instance, you might switch from gardening with a shovel to using raised garden beds for easier access.

Embrace Teamwork: Don't be afraid to ask for help! Work with your occupational therapist to develop strategies for adapting your hobbies or enlist the support of family and friends to assist you with certain tasks.

Overcoming Challenges and Maintaining Motivation

Adapting to new ways of doing things can be frustrating. Here are some tips to overcome challenges and maintain motivation:

Start Small and Celebrate Progress: Begin with short, achievable tasks and gradually increase the complexity as your skills and stamina improve. Celebrate every victory, no matter how small.

Focus on the Joy, Not Perfection: Remember, the goal is to enjoy your hobbies, not achieve perfection. Don't be discouraged by setbacks. Focus on the enjoyment and satisfaction you derive from the activity.

Join a Support Group: Connecting with others who have faced similar challenges can be a source of encouragement and inspiration. Support groups can offer practical tips and shared experiences to help you stay motivated.

Embrace Patience: Recovering from a stroke and adapting your hobbies takes time. Be patient with yourself and allow yourself the time and space to adjust and rediscover your passions.

Adapting your hobbies after a stroke is not about giving up; it's about finding new ways to engage in the activities you love. By embracing creativity, seeking support, and focusing on the joy of participation, you can reignite your passions and continue to experience the fulfillment and satisfaction your hobbies bring to your life.

10.3 Finding Meaning and Purpose After Stroke

A stroke can be a life-altering event, disrupting your routines, impacting your abilities, and leaving you questioning your purpose and place in the world. During your recovery journey, it's natural to grapple with feelings of loss and uncertainty. However, a stroke doesn't define your worth or diminish your capacity to live a meaningful and fulfilling life. This chapter explores the importance of finding purpose after a stroke, offers strategies for reshaping your narrative, and emphasizes the power of embracing a life filled with purpose and contribution.

The Search for Meaning After a Stroke

The human spirit craves meaning. After a stroke, the search for meaning can feel particularly profound. Here's why finding purpose is crucial for a fulfilling life after a stroke:

Provides Direction and Motivation: A sense of purpose gives direction to your life and fuels your motivation to engage in activities and strive for goals.

Enhances Well-Being: Living with purpose fosters feelings of self-worth, accomplishment, and satisfaction, contributing to overall well-being.

Promotes Resilience: When you have a sense of purpose, it empowers you to navigate challenges and setbacks with greater resilience.

Connects You to Others: Finding purpose often involves contributing to something larger than yourself. This fosters connection and builds a sense of belonging within your community.

Reshaping Your Narrative

After a stroke, it's easy to fall into a narrative of loss and limitation. However, this narrative doesn't have to define your future. Here's how to reshape your story and find meaning after a stroke:

Focus on What You Can Do: Shift your mindset. Instead of dwelling on what you've lost, focus on your remaining abilities and the new skills you're developing through rehabilitation.

Redefine Your Goals: Your goals might need to adjust after a stroke, but new goals can be just as fulfilling. Consider what brings you joy and what you want to achieve in this new chapter of your life.

Embrace New Challenges: Don't be afraid to step outside your comfort zone. Learning new skills, volunteering for a cause you care about, or pursuing a creative endeavor can inject meaning and purpose into your life.

Find Inspiration: Connect with others who have overcome similar challenges. Their stories of resilience and their pursuit of purpose can be a source of inspiration and motivation.

Celebrate Your Achievements: Acknowledge and celebrate your progress, no matter how small. Every step forward towards living a meaningful life is a victory.

By focusing on what you can do, setting new goals, embracing challenges, seeking inspiration, and celebrating your achievements, you can reshape your narrative. Remember, a stroke is a part of your story, but it doesn't define your whole life. Embrace this opportunity to find new purpose and continue to lead a fulfilling and meaningful life.

CHAPTER ELEVEN

BUILDING EMOTIONAL RESILIENCE

11.1 COPING WITH FRUSTRATION AND DISCOURAGEMENT

The road to recovery after a stroke can be long and challenging. It's natural to feel frustrated and discouraged along the way. Whether it's dealing with physical limitations, struggling to regain lost skills, or facing setbacks, these negative emotions can be overwhelming. This chapter explores strategies for coping with frustration and discouragement after a stroke, provides tools for managing emotional challenges, and emphasizes the importance of building resilience for a successful recovery journey.

The Grip of Frustration and Discouragement

Frustration and discouragement are common emotions after a stroke. Understanding these feelings is crucial because:

They are Valid Responses: Given the challenges you face, it's normal to feel frustrated and discouraged. Acknowledge these emotions without judgment.

They Can Hinder Progress: If left unchecked, these negative emotions can drain your motivation and impede your progress in rehabilitation and daily life.

Strategies for Managing Frustration

Frustration can be a powerful emotion. Here are some tips to manage it effectively:

Identify Your Triggers: Recognize situations or activities that typically trigger your frustration. Once you identify them, you can develop strategies to cope.

Take a Deep Breath: When frustration arises, take a few deep breaths to calm your body and mind. Practice relaxation techniques like mindfulness meditation to manage these emotions.

Reframe Your Thinking: Challenge negative thoughts that contribute to frustration. Focus on the progress you've made, not what you haven't achieved yet.

Break Down Tasks: Large tasks can feel overwhelming and contribute to frustration. Break them down into smaller, more manageable steps. Completing these smaller tasks can provide a sense of accomplishment and boost your mood.

Focus on the Positive: Make a conscious effort to focus on the positive aspects of your recovery journey. Celebrate your successes, no matter how small.

Combating Discouragement

Discouragement can sap your motivation. Here are some strategies to combat it:

Set Realistic Goals: Unrealistic goals can set you up for disappointment. Work with your doctor and rehabilitation team to set achievable goals that celebrate progress.

Focus on Progress, Not Perfection: Recovery is a journey, not a destination. Don't be discouraged by setbacks. Focus on the progress you've made and trust that continued effort will yield further improvement.

Reward Yourself: Celebrating milestones, no matter how small, can boost your motivation and keep you moving forward. Reward yourself for completing tasks or achieving goals.

Maintain a Positive Attitude: Developing a positive mindset is crucial. Focus on what you can control and approach challenges with optimism and determination.

Seek Support: Don't hesitate to seek support from your loved ones, therapists, or a support group. Talking about your discouragement can help you process these emotions and build resilience.

Building Resilience for Long-Term Success

Resilience is the ability to bounce back from setbacks and challenges. Here are some ways to cultivate resilience on your recovery journey:

Practice Self-Compassion: Be kind to yourself. Recovery takes time and effort. Don't beat yourself up for setbacks or moments of frustration.

Maintain a Strong Support System: Surround yourself with positive and supportive people who believe in you and your ability to recover.

Focus on Healthy Habits: Prioritize good sleep, healthy eating, and regular exercise. These habits promote physical and mental well-being, which in turn strengthens your resilience.

Find Meaning and Purpose: Having a sense of purpose in life can be a powerful motivator and can help you weather challenges with greater strength.

Celebrate Your Strength: Acknowledge your inner strength and resilience. Remember, you've already overcome a major challenge – the stroke itself. You have the strength to navigate the challenges of recovery.

By understanding and addressing frustration and discouragement, and by building resilience, you can continue to move forward on your recovery journey. Remember, every step forward, no matter how small, is a victory.

11.2 Managing Anxiety and Depression After Stroke

The aftermath of a stroke can bring immense emotional turmoil. Anxiety and depression are common emotional responses that can significantly impact your recovery. This chapter explores the signs and symptoms of anxiety and depression after a stroke, offers strategies for managing these conditions, and underscores the importance of seeking professional help when needed.

Understanding Anxiety and Depression After Stroke

Anxiety: This is characterized by excessive worry, fear, and physical symptoms like rapid heartbeat, shortness of breath, and muscle tension. After a stroke, anxiety can stem from concerns about your health, regaining abilities, and the future.

Depression: This manifests as feelings of sadness, hopelessness, loss of interest in activities you once enjoyed, and changes in sleep or appetite. These feelings can be triggered by the limitations imposed by the stroke, impacting your self-esteem and sense of purpose.

Recognizing the Signs and Symptoms

It's crucial to recognize the signs and symptoms of anxiety and depression after a stroke. Here are some common indicators:

ANXIETY:

- Constant worry or fear
- Difficulty concentrating
- Irritability
- Difficulty sleeping
- Panic attacks

DEPRESSION:

- Feeling sad or down most of the time
- Loss of interest in pleasurable activities
- Changes in appetite or weight
- Sleep problems (sleeping too much or too little)

- Feelings of worthlessness or guilt

- Difficulty thinking clearly or making decisions

- Thoughts of death or suicide

Note: These are just some common signs and symptoms. If you are experiencing any of these issues, it's important to speak with your doctor or a mental health professional for a proper diagnosis.

Strategies for Managing Anxiety and Depression

Here are some strategies to help manage anxiety and depression after a stroke:

Talk Therapy: Cognitive Behavioral Therapy (CBT) can be highly effective. It helps you identify negative thought patterns and develop coping mechanisms to manage them.

Medication: Sometimes medication is helpful in managing anxiety and depression. Discuss treatment options with your doctor to determine the best approach for you.

Relaxation Techniques: Practices like deep breathing exercises, mindfulness meditation, and progressive muscle relaxation can help reduce anxiety and promote calm.

Healthy Lifestyle Habits: Maintaining a healthy sleep routine, engaging in regular exercise, and eating a balanced diet can significantly improve your mood and reduce stress levels.

Social Connection: Spending time with loved ones, joining a support group, or engaging in social activities can combat feelings of isolation and loneliness, which can contribute to anxiety and depression.

When to Seek Professional Help

If your symptoms of anxiety or depression are severe, interfere with your daily life, or persist despite your efforts to manage them, it's crucial to seek professional help. Here are some signs that indicate professional intervention is **necessary:**

Thoughts of self-harm or suicide

Difficulty coping with daily activities

Excessive anxiety that interferes with sleep or work

Feelings of hopelessness or worthlessness

Loss of interest in activities you once enjoyed

Recognizing and addressing anxiety and depression after a stroke is essential for your overall well-being. By utilizing these strategies and seeking help when needed, you can better navigate your recovery journey.

11.3 Finding Hope and Building a Positive Outlook

The journey after a stroke can feel overwhelming, filled with limitations, uncertainties, and emotional challenges that may cast a shadow of discouragement. However, hope is a powerful force that can light your path and fuel your recovery. This chapter explores the importance of fostering hope and cultivating a positive outlook after a stroke. We will delve into strategies for nurturing optimism, reframing negative thoughts, and embracing a future filled with possibility.

The Power of Hope After Stroke

Hope is more than just a wish for a better future. It's a belief in your ability to overcome challenges and a driving force that motivates you to move forward. Here's why fostering hope is crucial after a stroke:

Improves Emotional Well-Being: Hope counteracts feelings of despair and depression, promoting a more positive outlook and a sense of resilience.

Enhances Motivation: Believing in the possibility of recovery motivates you to engage in rehabilitation and persevere through setbacks.

Increases Focus: Hope helps you maintain focus on your goals and empowers you to take action towards achieving them.

Strengthens Resilience: A hopeful outlook allows you to bounce back from challenges and navigate the uncertainties of recovery with greater strength.

Cultivating a Positive Outlook

Building a positive outlook is an ongoing process. Here are some strategies to nurture optimism after a stroke:

Focus on Progress, Not Perfection: Recovery takes time. Celebrate your achievements, no matter how small, and acknowledge the progress you've made.

Challenge Negative Thoughts: Identify negative thoughts that might be holding you back. Challenge their validity and replace them with more realistic and empowering beliefs.

Practice Gratitude: Focus on the things you're grateful for—your loved ones, your support system, and even small victories in your recovery journey. Gratitude fosters a positive outlook.

Visualize Success: Spend time visualizing yourself achieving your recovery goals. Mental imagery can be a powerful tool for boosting optimism.

Surround Yourself with Positivity: Spend time with supportive and encouraging people who believe in you and your potential for recovery.

Finding Hope in Everyday Moments

Hope isn't a destination; it's a journey nurtured by everyday experiences. Here are some ways to find hope in your daily life:

Focus on Abilities: Shift your focus from what you can't do to what you can do. Explore your remaining abilities and find ways to utilize them in your daily life.

Connect with Others: Social interaction and building strong relationships can be a source of hope and support.

Engage in Activities You Enjoy: Participating in activities you find meaningful and enjoyable can bring joy and a sense of purpose back into your life.

Celebrate Milestones: No matter how small, acknowledge and celebrate your milestones along the way. These celebrations reinforce your progress and keep you motivated.

Embrace the Power of Inspiration: Read stories of others who have overcome challenges after a stroke. Their resilience and determination can be a source of hope and inspiration for your own journey.

Hope is a powerful force that can transform your recovery journey, helping you navigate the challenges and uncertainties of life after a stroke. By cultivating a positive outlook and finding hope in everyday moments, you can embrace a future filled with possibility and resilience.

CHAPTER TWELVE

RETURNING TO WORK AND SOCIAL ACTIVITIES

12.1 CONSIDERATIONS FOR RETURNING TO WORK

Returning to work after experiencing a stroke is a decision that involves careful consideration of various factors. This chapter explores the complexities surrounding this decision, provides strategies for successful workplace reintegration, and underscores the importance of open communication and collaboration with both your employer and healthcare team.

Returning to Work After Stroke:

Deciding whether to return to work post-stroke is deeply personal, with no one-size-fits-all answer. Here are some key factors to weigh:

Stroke Severity: The severity of your stroke and its impact on your abilities are significant factors influencing your decision.

Health Status: Consider your overall physical and cognitive health, energy levels, and any recommendations from your doctor.

Job Demands: Assess whether you can meet the physical and cognitive demands of your previous job, with or without modifications.

Emotional Readiness: Returning to work can be emotionally challenging. Reflect on your emotional well-being and readiness for the workplace environment.

Financial Considerations: Evaluate your financial situation and explore options like part-time work, disability benefits, or career retraining.

Planning for a Successful Reintegration:

Should you choose to return to work, thorough planning is essential. Here are some strategies to ensure a smooth transition:

Open Communication: Discuss your stroke, limitations, and potential modifications with your employer openly and honestly.

Collaboration with Healthcare Team: Work with your healthcare professionals to create a return-to-work plan, including workplace modifications or a phased return schedule.

Explore Accommodations: Investigate accommodations your employer can provide, as they're often required by law for employees with disabilities.

Retraining Options: If returning to your previous job isn't feasible, explore retraining opportunities for a new career path that suits your abilities and interests.

Open Communication is Key:

Maintaining open communication throughout the process is crucial. Here are some communication tips:

Clarity and Transparency: Clearly communicate your limitations and needs to your employer and colleagues.

Self-Advocacy: Advocate for the accommodations or modifications necessary for your success in the workplace.

Ongoing Dialogue: Keep the lines of communication open with both your employer and healthcare team as your needs may change over time.

Navigating a return to work after a stroke requires thoughtful consideration, strategic planning, and effective communication. By addressing these aspects proactively, you can increase the likelihood of a successful transition back into the workforce.

12.2 Adapting Your Work Environment for Success

Returning to work post-stroke can feel overwhelming as you navigate challenges in your familiar workplace. However, with a focus on accessibility and collaboration, you can adapt your work environment to support your success. This chapter explores strategies for creating an accessible workspace, considering potential modifications, and advocating for your needs positively and collaboratively.

Creating an Accessible Workspace:

Making your workspace accessible is essential. Here's how:

Ergonomics: Ensure ergonomic equipment like adjustable chairs and keyboards to minimize physical discomfort.

Lighting: Optimize lighting to reduce eye strain and enhance visibility.

Noise Reduction: Use noise-cancelling headphones or seek a quiet workspace if noise is a distraction.

Assistive Technologies: Explore tools like screen readers or voice recognition software to aid in your tasks effectively.

Exploring Workplace Modifications:

Consider modifications tailored to your needs:

Physical Modifications: Adjust your workspace layout or furniture to accommodate physical limitations.

Schedule Adjustments: Discuss flexible work hours or phased returns to manage energy levels.

Task Modifications: Simplify tasks, delegate, or utilize assistive technologies.

Communication Support: Use aids or additional time for processing information during meetings.

The Power of Collaboration and Advocacy:

Advocate for your needs in a collaborative manner:

Focus on Solutions: Present modifications as solutions to enhance job performance.

Provide Documentation: Obtain recommendations from healthcare professionals to support your requests.

Highlight Your Strengths: Emphasize your skills and value as an employee.

Maintain Positivity: Approach discussions positively to foster productive dialogue.

Be Specific: Clearly communicate your needs and desired modifications.

Finding Support and Resources:

Explore available resources for assistance:

Vocational Rehabilitation Services: Government agencies offer services to help assess skills and develop return-to-work plans.

Disability Rights Organizations: Seek information and advocacy support regarding workplace rights.

Employer Assistance Programs: Utilize programs that offer resources for navigating challenges post-stroke.

Advocating for your needs and collaborating with your employer can create an empowering work environment post-stroke. In the next chapter, we'll discuss building a robust support system to aid in your recovery journey, covering communication strategies with loved ones and fostering a supportive network.

12.3 Reconnecting with Friends, Family, and the Community

Recovering from a stroke can sometimes leave you feeling disconnected from your social life, but rebuilding those connections is crucial for your well-being. This chapter explores why social connection matters, offers strategies for reconnecting with loved ones, and suggests ways to engage with your community.

The Importance of Social Connection After Stroke:

Here's why social connection matters:

Reduces Loneliness: Being socially connected can combat feelings of loneliness and isolation, which are common after a stroke.

Boosts Well-being: Spending time with loved ones and engaging in social activities can make you feel happier and more fulfilled.

Provides Support: Your social circle can offer practical assistance and emotional support as you navigate your recovery journey.

Enhances Quality of Life: Social interaction adds meaning to your life and contributes to an overall better quality of life.

Rebuilding Your Social Circle:

Reconnecting with loved ones takes effort. Here's how to do it:

Initiate Contact: Reach out to friends and family through calls, texts, or video chats.

Communicate Openly: Be honest about your stroke, limitations, and emotional needs.

Set Realistic Expectations: Take your time getting back into social activities and don't pressure yourself to do too much too soon.

Find New Ways to Connect: Get creative with virtual gatherings like game nights or movie marathons to maintain social interaction.

Effective Communication with Loved Ones:

Communication is key. Here's how to communicate effectively:

Be Clear and Direct: Clearly express your needs and don't hesitate to ask for support.

Practice Patience: Understand that adjusting to your new reality takes time for both you and your loved ones.

Listen Actively: Pay attention to what others are saying and acknowledge their concerns.

Focus on the Positive: Share your progress and focus on creating enjoyable experiences together.

Finding New Ways to Connect with Your Community:

Getting involved in your community can provide support and purpose. Here's how:

Support Groups: Join a stroke support group to connect with others who understand what you're going through.

Community Centers: Explore activities or volunteering opportunities offered by local community centers.

Online Communities: Participate in online forums or groups where you can connect with fellow stroke survivors.

Remember,

Rebuilding your social circle is a process. Be patient with yourself and celebrate every step forward. With open communication, a positive attitude, and a willingness to explore new ways to connect, you can build a strong support network that enriches your life after stroke.

CONCLUSION

The journey after a stroke isn't a sprint; it's more like a marathon. There will be tough moments, setbacks that shake your confidence, and days clouded with uncertainty. But deep within you lies a well of resilience, a strength waiting to be tapped. This book has armed you with tools and strategies to navigate this journey – to handle frustration, nurture hope, and rebuild your life with purpose.

Think about John, the carpenter you met at the support group. Despite never fully regaining the use of his right arm after his stroke two years ago, he found innovative ways to adapt his craft. With a specially designed brace and jigs, he continues woodworking, crafting beautiful pieces that inspire others. John's story shows the power of resilience and the ability to thrive despite limitations.

Then there's Sarah, the lively artist who faced a stroke affecting her speech. Though she sometimes struggles to find words, her creativity hasn't waned. Through painting, sketching, and assistive technology, she creates stunning visual art that speaks volumes. Sarah's journey underscores the human spirit's capacity to find alternative paths to expression and live a creatively rich life.

Your story will mirror resilience, adaptation, and rediscovery. There will be days when progress feels sluggish and limitations loom large. On those days, draw strength from John, Sarah, and countless others who've trodden this path. Remember the tools you've gained:

Focus on possibilities, not limitations. John found ways to work around his weakened arm.

Maintain a positive outlook. Sarah's optimism fueled her creativity and resourcefulness.

Seek support and foster a strong network. Both John and Sarah found solace and encouragement in their support groups.

The road ahead may twist and turn, but a fulfilling life brimming with purpose is within reach. Prioritize your well-being, nurture your passions, and seize the growth opportunities in this new chapter. Challenges will come, but with steadfast determination and the love of your dear ones, you can craft a life that's meaningful, vibrant, and uniquely yours.

This book is just the beginning. Carry its lessons, face challenges with courage, and celebrate every victory. Remember, you're not alone on this journey. With resilience and hope, you can forge a future filled with promise after a stroke.

"Thanks for reading! If you enjoyed this book or found it useful, I'd be very grateful if you'd post a short review on Amazon. Your support really does make a difference and I read all the reviews personally so I can get your feedback and make this book even better.